£20.80

Medical Receptionists and Secretaries Handbook

Third edition

Mari Robbins

Radcliffe Medical Press

Radcliffe Medical Press Ltd
18 Marcham Road
Abingdon
Oxon OX14 1AA
United Kingdom

www.radcliffe-oxford.com
The Radcliffe Medical Press electronic catalogue and online ordering facility.
Direct sales to anywhere in the world.

British Library Cataloguing in Publication Data

A catalogue record for this book is available from the British Library.

ISBN 1 85775 565 0

Typeset by AMA DataSet Limited, Preston, Lancs
Printed and bound by TJ International Ltd, Padstow, Cornwall

Contents

Preface

The success of the previous editions of this book, first published in 1996, has been responsible for the opportunity to write a third edition of the *Medical Receptionists and Secretaries Handbook*.

Once again, the new edition is published at a time of ever-escalating changes in the National Health Service, which is embarking once more on a journey of extensive reforms. As a result, managers, with the support of their receptionists and secretaries, are facing the task of implementing the NHS Plan, which affects all areas of primary and secondary healthcare.

The third edition has enabled me to incorporate changes which have taken place since 1998, but also to include sections on issues that reflect the rapid changes taking place within the health service as the NHS Plan is implemented. These changes affect all members of healthcare teams. The chapter on private medicine has been further expanded to include the change in the relationship between the NHS and the private sector, the introduction of clinical governance, and the regulation of independent hospitals – a challenge for all who work in this sector.

Times of change are never easy, and professionals, their healthcare teams and patients tend to mistrust changes to their services. It is therefore important that all those involved in the provision and delivery of healthcare should have an understanding of what the changes involve, and work as a team to ensure that both the National Health Service and the private sector will achieve improved and effective health and social care based on identified patient needs.

More than ever the medical receptionist and secretary will provide the vital link between patients and providers of healthcare within the national and private sectors.

Mari Robbins
November 2001

Contributor

Sally Storey
Director of Human Resources
Bournewood Community and Mental Health NHS Trust
Guildford Road
Chertsey
KT16 0QA

Acknowledgements

My acknowledgements and sincere thanks go to Richard Fryer, Manager of the Old Coulsdon Medical Practice, Old Coulsdon, Sue Dunlop, Secretary to Mr MA Edgar, Harley Street, London, Ivan Chu, Health and Safety Adviser, Bournewood Community and Mental Health Trust and Barbara Stewart.

In revising material for this edition, I have found both the NHS and the Department of Health websites an invaluable source of current information.

The National Health Service

History

Prior to the National Health Service Act of 1946, healthcare in the UK had developed in an ad hoc manner.

The medical profession had, since the latter part of the nineteenth century, gradually acquired social respectability, legal status and economic strength. The concept of public responsibility for the health of individuals can be traced back to 1834, when the Poor Law Amendment Act was passed, which established that parish workhouses should provide sick wards where the able-bodied inhabitants could be treated when they became unwell. However, as the health of the community had been severely neglected, it became necessary for the workhouses to admit the sick paupers from the parish to their wards – people who had hitherto been left to die as they were unable to obtain medical care themselves. By 1848 the demand for institutional care was such that the sick wards of the workhouses had become entirely devoted to sick paupers. The Public Health Act of that year acknowledged for the first time the State's responsibility for institutional care.

The quality of medical care available improved as scientists made important discoveries. Florence Nightingale, in her contribution to both nurse training and hospital planning, revolutionised the standards of institutional care. Largely due to the philanthropy of the well-to-do and the moral obligations of the charitable and religious bodies, the end of the nineteenth century heralded the opening of many voluntary and private hospitals. Voluntary hospitals were financed through subscriptions and donations, and attracted the services of skilled doctors, some of whom, acting on their social conscience, often treated patients without payment.

The beginning of the twentieth century saw the advent of insurance schemes which enabled individuals to protect themselves against sickness and injuries which might involve them in expensive medical care or affect their capacity to work.

However, despite the progress that was being made, the standard of medical and nursing care emerging throughout the country was inconsistent in both quality and availability.

At the end of the First World War, the first Ministry of Health was established, which together with various reforms provided the stimulus for a nationally organised health service. The Second World War brought about further reforms and the publishing of the Beveridge Report in 1942 with its recommendations that formed the basis for the post-war system of social welfare services, and the provision of a comprehensive system of healthcare. Sir William Beveridge recommended that the term 'comprehensive' meant that medical treatment should be available for every citizen, both in the home and in hospital, and provided by general practitioners, specialist physicians and surgeons, dentists, opticians, nurses and midwives. He also advocated the provision of surgical appliances and rehabilitation services.

Thus the National Health Service (NHS) became effective in 1948, with the aim of improving the health of the people, providing healthcare through a system of public finance and public provision and, by eradicating disease, reducing the demand for free healthcare services. The NHS took over all hospitals, convalescent homes and rehabilitation units, offering consultants contracts as full-time salaried employees. General medical practitioners providing family doctor services were encouraged to sign contracts to provide family practitioner services for patients in their area, and were permitted to remain self-employed but paid by the health service on a fee basis.

Medical services fell into the following three functional areas:

- those concerned with the sick person in the community

- those concerned with the sick person in an institution

- those concerned with preventive medical services.

They were identified with the following services:

- general practitioner services

- hospital services

- services provided by the local authority (excluding school health services).

The hospital service was administered by regional hospital boards, which absorbed all of the public and voluntary hospitals in the country. The national planning of hospital requirements was established.

Teaching hospitals in England and Wales remained relatively independent with their boards of governors who were responsible directly to the

Secretary of State, but they were linked only to the regional hospital boards in that there was one teaching hospital in each region.

General practitioner services were organised through executive councils, which administered the family doctors' contracts and dental, pharmaceutical and ophthalmic services. The local health authorities administered the preventive services, ambulance services, etc.

The main advantage of the NHS was that it had brought together services which had previously been under the control of independent organisations. However, administration of this tripartite arrangement was far from satisfactory, and in an attempt to improve the co-ordination of healthcare between hospital boards, local executive councils and the type of care provided by local authorities, the 1974 National Health Service Reorganisation Act came into force.

Reorganising the NHS

The 1974 reorganisation brought about changes in the way in which the NHS was organised and structured, including the following:

- the formation of regional health authorities (RHAs)

- the formation of area health authorities (AHAs) with directly accountable districts

- community healthcare, which hitherto had been the responsibility of local authorities, moved to the NHS

- executive councils were abolished and replaced by family practitioner committees (FPCs) to administer family practitioner services (general medical, dental and ophthalmic services, and the pharmaceutical services provided by retail pharmacists).

The changes introduced to the NHS the concept of planning and improvement in personnel and manpower controls.

Two issues that arose from this reorganisation and which remain today were the creation of the following:

- community health councils

- health service commissioner.

Community health councils

Community health councils (CHCs) were created with the 1974 reorganisation (generally one for each health district), to represent the interests of the people in their community. Their main function is to make constructive criticisms and recommendations to the health authorities on the provision of services in their district. They also advise patients on how they may make complaints about the services.

Health service commissioner (Ombudsman)

Another feature arising from the 1974 reorganisation was the appointment of the health service commissioner to investigate complaints within the NHS, giving complainants direct access to the commissioner. The commissioner will not investigate a complaint unless he or she is satisfied that the health authority concerned has had a reasonable opportunity to look into and reply to the complaint. Initially, the commissioner could not investigate areas covering family practitioner matters, but since April 1996 the proposals for a new complaints procedure, outlined in *Acting on Complaints*, confirmed that the Government would legislate to extend the jurisdiction of the health service commissioner to all complaints by or on behalf of NHS patients. The legislation brings within the Ombudsman's power complaints about the following:

- NHS services provided by family health services practitioners, their staff or deputies or locums

- actions taken wholly or partly as a result of the exercise of clinical judgement.

The Ombudsman is completely independent of the NHS and the Government. As well as complaints about the NHS services, he or she can investigate complaints about how the complaints procedure is working.

The Ombudsman is not obliged to investigate every complaint, and will not generally take on a case which has not first been through the NHS complaints procedure.

The 1982 reorganisation

The aims of this restructuring were as follows:

- simplification

- the strengthening of local-level management.

The restructuring was intended to deliver greater efficiency and accountability of the service to Parliament, including the direct responsibility of the Family Practitioner Committees to the Secretary of State and greater responsibility for managing their own affairs (*see* Figure 1.1).

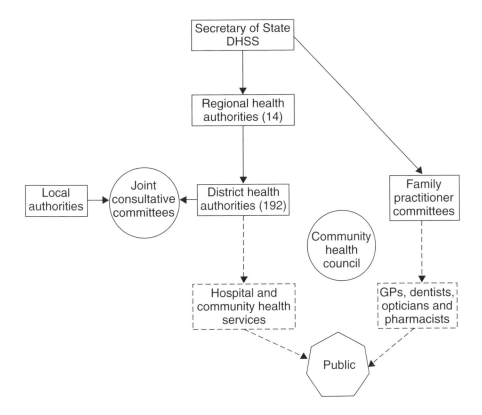

Figure 1.1   The NHS reorganisation in England in 1984.

The changing NHS

In the early 1990s, the NHS experienced a programme of reforms that was more extensive and fundamental than any reorganisation since its inception. The changes arose from proposals made in the following three White Papers:

- *Promoting Better Health* (1987)
- *Working for Patients* (1989)
- *Caring for People* (1989).

The Government stated that the proposal for reforms would not affect the basic principles of the NHS to provide:

> a comprehensive health service designed to secure improvement in the physical and mental health of the people of England and Wales, and the prevention, diagnosis and treatment of illness.

The reforms required certain statutory changes, and these were embodied in the 1990 NHS and Community Care Act.

The most important of these reforms were as follows:

- the introduction of a new system of contractual funding

- measures to manage clinical activity more effectively

- proposals to strengthen management at all levels

- new arrangements for allocating resources.

The NHS reforms and changes were intended to tackle the underlying problems in management and funding of the health service. By introducing competition between providers of health services in the form of an 'internal market', the Government intended to increase the efficiency and effectiveness with which resources were used. Services would also be more responsive to users by giving them greater choice. Providers of health services were encouraged to become NHS trusts, taking greater control over the management of their own affairs, including greater freedom to raise capital and to determine staffing structures and rates of pay. The 'purchasers' in this internal market would be either district health authorities (DHAs) or GP fundholders (GPFHs).

The organisation of the National Health Service in the early 1990s

The basic structure of the NHS in England following the 1990 reforms is shown in Figure 1.2.

Community health councils and patient empowerment

Community health councils (CHCs) are statutory bodies that were established in 1974 to represent the interest of the public in local health provision and to act as a channel for consumer concerns. It was agreed that CHCs should have the following rights:

- to relevant information from local NHS authorities, PCGs and trusts

- to access certain NHS premises

- to inclusion in consultation on substantial developments or variations in local health services in hospitals and in the community

- to send observers to meetings of health authorities and trusts

- to act as a channel for complaints or problems encountered by patients.

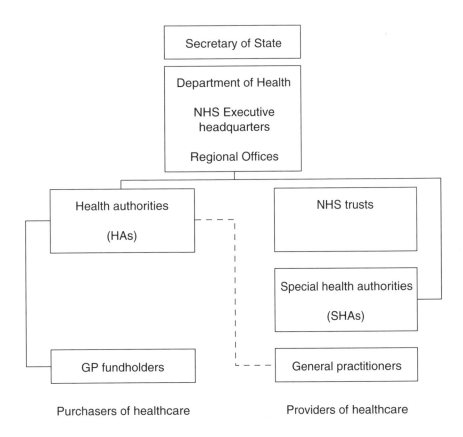

Figure 1.2 Structure of the NHS (*Source*: NHS Executive).

Many CHCs have accepted the need for change and indeed have been pushing the Government to make decisions. Despite the many significant changes to the NHS, CHCs have remained largely unchanged since they were set up. Their performance, it is widely accepted, is patchy and the services they provide are variable. In addition, CHCs have no rights within primary care – a huge disadvantage considering 70% of all patient contact is through primary care.

In reflection of these concerns, the NHS Plan set out the Government's ambitions to create a patient-centred NHS, and to move away from an outdated system of patients being on the outside, towards a new model where the voices of patients, their carers and the public are heard through every level of the service, acting as a powerful lever for change and improvement.

The findings of the Bristol inquiry have added impetus to these changes. Professor Kennedy's inquiry into the Bristol Royal Infirmary set out the principles which should lead to greater public and patient empowerment. The Government accepted these principles, and has developed proposals for reform to ensure that these are acted upon throughout the NHS.

The principles underpinning public and patient empowerment as set out in the Kennedy Report are as follow:

- patients and the public are entitled to be involved wherever decisions are taken about care in the NHS

- the involvement of patients and the public must be embedded in the structures of the NHS and permeate all aspects of healthcare

- the public and patients should have access to relevant information

- healthcare professionals must be partners in the process of involving the public and patients

- there must be honesty about the scope of the public's and patients' involvement, since some decisions cannot be made by the public

- there must be transparency and openness in the procedures for involving the public and patients

- the mechanisms for involvement should be evaluated for their effectiveness

- the public and patients should have access to training and funding to allow them to participate fully

- the public should be represented by a wide range of individuals and groups and not by particular 'patient groups'.

The Government is currently consulting on its intention to legislate at the earliest opportunity to replace CHCs with a set of arrangements that will:

- align the structures for patient and public involvement with the devolution of resources and power to the NHS frontline as outlined in *Shifting the Balance of Power within the NHS*

- integrate the views of patients and citizens into every level of the NHS, and ensure that involvement and support is consistent throughout

- make it easier to listen to patients' voices across the NHS so that services reflect their needs

- make it easier for citizens to contribute to strategic decisions so that services reflect and meet the needs of communities.

Patient Advocacy and Liaison Service (PALS)

A Patient Advocacy and Liaison Service is to be set up in every trust by 2002 as a result of the NHS Plan, to resolve complaints and concerns of patients quickly. They will act as an independent facilitator to handle patient or family concerns with direct access to the chief executive, and power to negotiate immediate solutions. PALS will be linked to the wider Patients' Forum for the locality. The Patients' Forum will be a statutory organisation independent of the trust. Patients' Forum members will be appointed through the NHS Appointments Commission, which is independent of the Secretary of State.

Purchaser/provider split and the internal market

Since 1991 the responsibilities for determining what healthcare is needed by the population and purchasing accordingly from a range of providers have been separated from those of providing hospital and community health services. This development of an 'internal market' was intended to address a range of problems, such as growing waiting-lists, which had arisen during the 1980s as demand for services increased.

Health authorities were established to commission (i.e. buy) the services needed by their local population from NHS trusts and other providers, including those in the independent sector.

Family health services authorities, in close liaison with health authorities, were responsible for planning and developing services to primary care in order to meet local needs. They became reorganised into the following categories.

Primary care groups (PCGs) are composed of GP practices, nurses and other community groups with an interest in primary care. PCGs became operational on 1 April 1999 when GP fundholding was abolished. All general practitioners are covered by the PCG in their locality. The role of PCGs is to contribute to the health improvement programme (HImP) and commission services within the HImP parameters, and in general to develop primary care locally. They work with other organisations to improve the health of a local area and work with social services to develop integrated health services.

Primary care trusts All primary care groups will eventually become primary care trusts (PCTs). PCTs shape local health and social health services. Their role is to bring about local health improvement, develop primary and community health services and commission hospital services.

GP fundholding was abolished in 2000 except in Northern Ireland, where it continues to expand. GP fundholders had their own budget to purchase some non-emergency hospital treatments and community health services for their patients (e.g. hip replacements, surgery, hernia operations, cataract operations, etc.).

Most NHS hospitals and community units became NHS trusts, providing services to health authorities and other purchasers on a contractual basis.

Observers credit the internal market with improved cost-consciousness in the NHS, but 'at a price' in that the competition which it encouraged between providers saw unnecessary duplication of services.

Patients of GP fundholders were often able to obtain treatment more quickly than patients of non-fundholders. This led to accusations of the NHS operating a two-tier system, contrary to the founding principles of the NHS of fair and equal access for all to healthcare.

The election of a new Government in May 1997 brought a new approach to the NHS. Pledging itself to the abolition of the internal market, the new Government set out an approach which aimed to build on what had worked previously, while discarding what had failed.

A new White Paper issued by the Department of Health, entitled *The New NHS: Modern, Dependable*, put forward a 'third way' of running the service that was based on partnership and driven by performance. The paper set out an approach which promised 'to go with the grain' of efforts by NHS staff to overcome obstacles within the internal market, building on the changes which had already taken place in the NHS to move away from outright competition and towards a more collaborative approach.

Six principles

The White Paper described the approach as a new model for the twenty-first century based on six key principles:

- to renew the NHS as a genuinely national service, offering fast access to consistently high-quality, prompt and accessible services across the country

- to make the delivery of healthcare against these new national standards a matter of local responsibility with local conditions, and with nurses 'in the driving seat' with regard to shaping services

- to get the NHS to work in partnership

- to drive efficiency through a more rigorous approach to performance, cutting bureaucracy to maximise every pound spent in the NHS for the care of patients

- to shift the focus on to quality of care so that excellence would be guaranteed to all patients, with quality as the driving force for decision making at every level of the service

- to rebuild confidence in the NHS as a public service that is account-able to patients, open to the public and shaped by their views.

The Health of the Nation

The Health of the Nation, which was published in 1992, provided an outline of the intended national health strategy which focused on health outcomes as well as healthcare, and which selected 'key' areas for action. It set national objectives and targets in these key areas, outlined initiatives to implement the action, and set out the framework for measuring, monitoring, development and review of key areas. This has now been overtaken by other measures.

The Patient's Charter

Published in 1992, the Patient's Charter was the NHS version of the Government's 'Citizen's Charter' initiative. It set out clear standards of service and emphasised quality of care, patient choice and the right to access to services, including receiving healthcare on the basis of clinical needs. Health authorities were encouraged to add their own local standards, and were held to account by the Department of Health for the publication of local charters and performance against certain standards. In 1995 this document was replaced by an expanded and updated Charter which responded to views expressed by patients and introduced new standards.

The NHS Plan commits to replacing the Patient's Charter with a new NHS Charter in 2001. It will clarify how people can access NHS services, the nature of the NHS commitment to patients, and the rights and responsibilities of patients within the NHS.

Quality of services

An important NHS goal is to improve the quality of services to individual patients, their carers and the wider community. One concern of the NHS is to ensure that both the quality and standard of healthcare are consistent across the UK. In your own organisation you may be part of a team involved in customer-care training, or developing an improved patient complaints procedure. You have the privilege of being the patient's first point of contact with the clinical team, and you are in an ideal position to identify the non-clinical needs of the patient.

Audit

Clinical audit is the systematic and critical analysis of the quality of clinical care, including the procedures used for diagnosis, treatment and care, the associated resources, and the resulting outcome and quality of life for the patient (Policy Statement on the Development of Clinical Audit).

Clinical audit embraces the audit activity of all healthcare professionals, including doctors, nurses and other healthcare staff. Audit should:

- be professionally led
- be seen as part of an educational process
- form part of routine clinical care
- be based on setting standards
- yield results that help to improve the outcome of the quality of care
- involve management in the process and outcomes of audit
- be confidential at the individual patient or clinical level
- take into consideration the views of the patient and their carer
- be an important part of quality programmes.

Secretaries, receptionists and audit

Secretaries and receptionists play an important part in the process of patient care, through their administrative work and their contact with patients. They are often asked to participate in audit activity, for example:

- by recording the time at which each patient arrives at the surgery or clinic, and the actual time when they are seen by a doctor
- by attendance at audit meetings to discuss ways of improving standards.

Remember that the patient's viewpoint and opinion play an important part in audit, and both secretaries and receptionists are in a good position to hear this view expressed.

Further change

The Health and Social Care Bill

The Health and Social Care Bill was published just before Christmas 2000. It is a vital part of the modernisation of the NHS, particularly for primary care. The reforms include the extension of nurse prescribing, the abolition of CHCs, powers to establish care trusts, and powers which will allow the Secretary of State to dismiss non-employees and suspend employees, effectively giving the Health Secretary the ability to remove whole boards and replace non-executive directors and chairmen.

Development of care trusts

Central to the modernisation agenda of the NHS Plan and the National Service Frameworks is improvement and measurement of the patient experience, recognising a wider environment of rising consumer expectations with regard to public services. Despite the best intentions, service users often describe their encounter with health and social services as a series of assessments from different perspectives that result in care plans being prescribed along the demarcation lines between professions.

Partnership flexibilities in the 1999 Health Act increased the range of options for promoting the integration of services. Ministers regard care trusts as an important additional element in the new partnership armoury. There are two models of care trusts:

- an enhanced primary care trust, commissioning and providing health and social care
- a mental health and social care trust provider organisation.

Proposals to extend nurse prescribing

Doctors and dentists are currently the only health professionals who are able to prescribe medicines on the basis of their professional training rather than against written protocols.

However, it is felt that there is considerable scope both for benefiting patients and for reducing workload of doctors by giving prescribing rights to other health professionals.

The Health and Social Care Bill provides for enabling legislative changes that will not only allow increased nurse prescribing across the UK, but will also extend prescribing rights to other professional groups.

Purpose of care trusts

Care trusts will be important vehicles for modernising both social and healthcare, helping to ensure integrated services that are focused on the needs of patients and users. They are neither a takeover of local government by the NHS nor a takeover of the NHS by local government. They are intended not only to broaden the range of possible options for health and social services and to deliver integrated care that gives the best service to the people who depend on both, but also to lead to improvements in the quality of service delivery.

The formation of care trusts does not mean that the Health Act flexibilities cannot continue to be used in other settings and situations. The Government expects that local councils will continue to develop lead commissioning and integrated provision. This will often be the most sensible response to the needs of particular client groups which have significant social care components to their needs, as well as a wide range of needs.

The NHS Plan

The NHS Plan, which was published in July 2000, sets out a vision of a health service designed around the patient. It is a radical action plan for the next 10 years, describing measures to put patients and people at the heart of the health service, and promising a 6.3% increase in funding over five years to 2004.

The aims of the NHS Plan are as follows.

- The NHS will provide a universal service for all based on clinical need, not on ability to pay.

- The NHS will provide a comprehensive range of services.

- The NHS will shape its services around the needs and preferences of individual patients, their families and their carers.

- The NHS will respond to the different needs of different populations.

- The NHS will work continuously to improve quality services and to minimise errors.

- The NHS will support and value its staff. Public funding for healthcare will be devoted solely to NHS patients.

- The NHS will work together with others to ensure a seamless service for patients.

- The NHS will help to keep people healthy and will work to reduce health inequalities.

- The NHS will respect the confidentiality of individual patients, and will provide open access to information about services, treatment and performance.

The NHS Plan promises the following:

- more power and information to patients
- more hospitals and beds
- more doctors and nurses
- much shorter waiting-times for hospital and doctor appointments
- cleaner wards and better food and facilities in hospitals
- improved care for older people
- tougher standards for NHS organisations and better rewards for the best.

NHS Plan priorities

These are the largest changes to face the NHS since it was set up 50 years ago. Ensuring that they happen means that the Government has had to prioritise. It has decided to:

- target the diseases which are the biggest killers, such as cancer and heart disease

- pinpoint the changes that are most urgently needed to improve people's health and well-being, and deliver the modern, fair and convenient services that people want.

Modernisation Board

A Modernisation Board has been set up to lead the changes. It has an advisory role and consists of leading figures from healthcare institutions

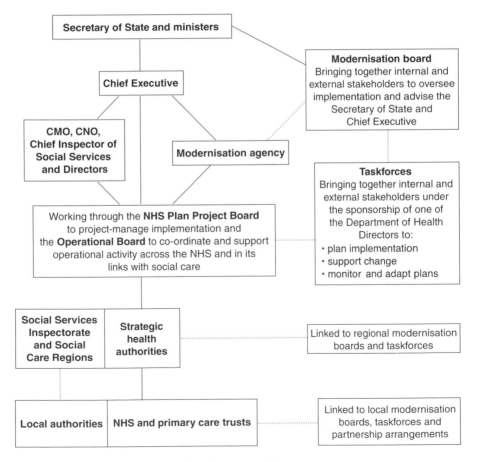

Figure 1.3   Summary of organisational structure plan.

such as the Royal Colleges, together with clinical staff and managers from within the NHS and patient representatives.

Taskforces

The Department of Health has to put in place ten taskforces to drive forward the ideas and improvements outlined in the plan.

Six of these taskforces will focus on 'what' services are being improved, namely:

- coronary heart disease

- cancer

- mental health

- older people

- children

- waiting-times and access to services.

The remaining four taskforces will concentrate on the following:

- the NHS workforce

- quality

- reducing inequalities and promoting public health

- investing in facilities and information technology.

Modernisation Agency

A new Modernisation Agency plays a critical role in ensuring that the commitments to the plan are translated into reality. The new agency will work with NHS trusts to help them to redesign their services around the needs and conveniences of patients.

The structure of the NHS

Department of Health

This is the Government department responsible for delivering a fast, fair, convenient and high-quality health and social care service to the people of England. The Department of Health has offices in Leeds and London. It is responsible for giving NHS organisations, such as hospital trusts and GPs, the information, guidance and support that they need in order to deliver the Government's policies and meet its standards of patient care.

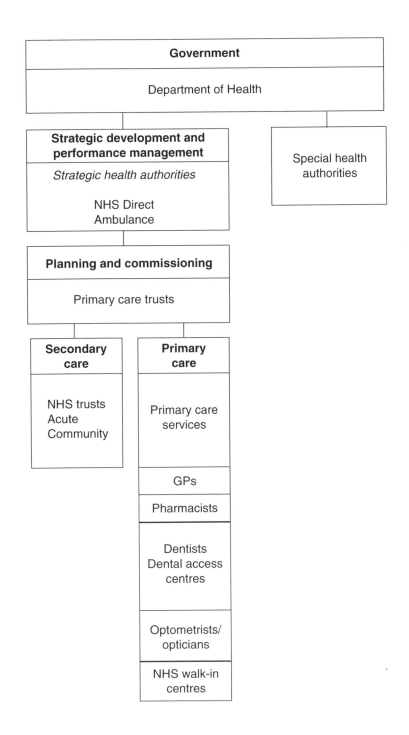

Figure 1.4 Structure of the National Health Service.

Strategic health authorities

In England, from April 2002, about 30 strategic health authorities will lead the strategic development of the local health service and performance manage PCTs and NHS trusts. These will replace the 98 health authorities. In Scotland this role is performed by the health boards, and in Northern Ireland it is the responsibility of the health and social services boards. A board of executive and non-executive directors runs each health authority. The non-executive directors are appointed by the Government. The executive directors are appointed by the chairperson of the authority, who is a non-executive member.

Primary care trusts

In April 2002, primary care trusts will become the lead NHS organisations in assessing need, planning and securing all health services and improving health. They will commission services from NHS trusts, as well as provide community-based services, and will monitor and manage performance against service agreements. PCTs will lead on the development of all primary care services, and will lead the NHS contribution to joint work with local government and other partners. They will be accountable to the Secretary of State through the strategic health authorities.

NHS Direct – 0845 4647

NHS Direct opened in March 1998 and offers fast and free 24-hour advice on personal healthcare. NHS Direct nurses aim to provide callers with the advice and reassurance which they need to care for themselves at home – or if they require further help, to direct them quickly to the right service at the right time. If a condition is more serious, or if it is an emergency, nurses can give quick advice on what action the caller should take and, if appropriate, will call an ambulance. Information and advice about the most common illnesses and a range of treatments is now also available on NHS Direct online (www.nhsdirect.nhs.uk).

NHS trusts

Hospital trusts are found in most large towns and cities, and usually offer a general range of secondary care and specialist services to meet most people's needs, working within delivery agreements with PCTs. Some trusts also act as regional or national centres of expertise for more specialised care, while some are attached to universities and help to train health professionals. Except in the case of emergencies, hospital treatment is arranged through general practitioners (i.e. by referral). Appointments and treatments are free. Together, NHS trusts employ the majority of the NHS workforce, including nurses, doctors, dentists, pharmacists, midwives, health visitors and staff from the professions allied to medicine, such as physiotherapists, radiographers, podiatrists, speech and language therapists, counsellors, occupational therapists and psychologists. Their many other staff include receptionists, secretaries, porters, cleaners, IT specialists and managers (*see* also Box 1.1).

Box 1.1 Types of trust

Primary care trusts
Primary care trusts are responsible for shaping local health and social care services. They are also responsible for commissioning secondary care services, and they provide and commission care and bring about local health improvement.

Acute hospital trusts
An acute trust provides a wide range of hospital-based treatments and services, and is usually situated near a district general hospital.

Community trusts
Community trusts are responsible for the provision of community services (e.g. district nursing, chiropody and home care services), and in some cases mental health services. They may also provide care for people with learning disabilities. Increasingly, primary care trusts are taking over these roles.

Mental health trusts
Mental health trusts are responsible for the provision of healthcare services to people with mental health problems. They may also provide care for people with learning disabilities.

Care trusts
Care trusts are a level of primary care trust with responsibilities for integrating primary care and social services provision. Legislation to enable their establishment is expected in 2002.

NHS walk-in centres

NHS walk-in centres offer fast access to health advice and treatment. They are open and available to anyone, and provide the following:

- a 7-day-a-week service
- assessment by an experienced NHS nurse
- treatment for minor injuries and illnesses
- instant access to health advice and information on other local services
- advice on how to stay healthy
- information on local out-of-hours GP and dental services
- information on pharmacy services.

The first NHS walk-in centres opened in January 2001, and there are now around 40 such centres.

Primary care

The first port of call for many people when they develop a health problem is their local general practitioner. These medical practitioners usually form a group practice that serves a particular neighbourhood. GPs are on the frontline of the NHS – primary care. Many other health professionals work as part of this frontline team, including nurses, health visitors, dentists, opticians, pharmacists and a range of specialist therapists. Every UK citizen has a right to be registered with a local GP, and visits to the surgery are free. NHS Direct and NHS walk-in centres are also part of primary care (*see also* Chapter 12 on primary healthcare services and social services).

Primary care groups (PCGs) and trusts (PCTs)

Since 1999, GPs have been able to join together to form 'primary care groups' along with other health professionals. This means that they are given the funding to work together to plan and commission health services for their local communities on behalf of health authorities. It also means that decisions about local services are made at a local level by those individuals who are best placed to make them. By April 2002, all PCGs will have been replaced by PCTs with formal responsibility for commissioning and providing health services.

Secondary care

Secondary care is specialised treatment, usually provided by a hospital.

Special health authorities

A special health authority is a health authority that provides health services to the whole population of England, and not just to a local community (e.g. the National Blood Authority).

Dental access centres

Dental access centres provide a complete range of NHS dental services, including routine as well as urgent care. People do not need to register to see a dentist in an access centre, and the centres are open at times when patients can get to them without inconvenience. The centres aim to improve access to dentistry. For details of your local dental access centre, contact NHS Direct.

General practitioners (GPs)

These are doctors who provide family health services to a local community. They are usually based in a surgery or GP practice, and they are often the first port of call for patients who are concerned about their health. GPs refer patients who need more help to specialists (e.g. hospital consultants).

Quality

The principle is that every part of the NHS and everyone who works in it should take responsibility for working to improve quality. This has to be quality in its broadest sense – doing the right things at the right time for the right people, and doing them right first time. It must cover the quality of the patient's experience as well as the clinical outcomes – quality measured in terms of prompt access, good relationships and efficient administration. This is achieved in the following three ways.

National level

National Service Frameworks (NSFs)

NSFs help to establish clear national standards for service to improve quality and reduce unacceptable variations in standards of care and treatment. There are NSFs for coronary heart disease, for mental health and for older people, as well as the NHS Cancer Plan. An NSF for diabetes is being developed.

National Institute for Clinical Excellence (NICE)

NICE is a new body that was set up in April 1999 to promote the highest quality of treatment and technology in the NHS and the cost-effectiveness of NHS services. It gives advice on best clinical practice in the NHS to those commissioning NHS services (health authorities and primary care groups/trusts), and to patients and their carers. NICE is a partnership between the Department of Health, the NHS, health professionals and patients. Guidelines set by NICE will be used across the country, helping to end the geographical variations in care that have developed in recent years.

National Clinical Assessment Authority (NCAA)

This new national body has been in operation since April 2001. It will provide a central point of contact for the NHS when concerns about a doctor's performance are raised. The authority will give advice to NHS hospitals and health authorities to ensure that the performance of doctors is checked and action is taken to ensure that doctors are practising safely. A report entitled *Assuring the Quality of Medical Practice* is available on the Internet, which provides details of this authority and other measures being taken to protect patients and support doctors.

Clinical governance

Clinical governance is a new statutory duty, which is intended to ensure that all patients receive quality healthcare. Doctors and other healthcare professionals in both primary and secondary care will take on a legal responsibility for standards of health service treatment.

Clinical governance brings together financial controls and good practice to improve performance. Quality will become an issue for everyone working in the NHS, both in clinical care and in management.

The main principles of clinical governance are as follows:

- an ability to identify easily where both responsibility and account-ability lie for the overall quality of medical care, wherever they are provided

- the use of a well-planned package of tools designed to improve the quality of health services, including clinical audit (which evaluates the results of treatment) and medical practice (which is based on research evidence and putting into place medical standards and guidelines)

- providing good staff education and training plans

- clear internal policies aimed at reducing the risk involved with any health service or medical treatment

- clear guidelines for self-regulation which can be applied to all profes-sional groups in order to identify and remedy poor performance.

Primary care groups and trusts, and NHS trusts are accountable for clinical governance and must ensure the quality of their health service and medical treatment.

Local level

Commission for Health Improvement (CHI)

The CHI will act as an independent inspectorate to ensure that the standards set by the Government through its health policies and NSFs and clinical guidance provided by NICE are met. Local care organisations in the NHS will be reviewed every three or four years. It also has the power to carry out or assist the following:

- *local primary care groups* which shape the services for their patients
- explicit *service standards* in local service agreements between health authorities, primary care groups/trusts and NHS trusts reflecting national standards and targets
- a new system of *clinical governance* in NHS trusts and primary care.

Efficiency

The NHS Plan set out six proposals to improve efficiency:

- clinical and financial responsibility united in new primary care groups responsible for a single unified budget covering most aspects of care
- limits imposed on management costs in health authorities and primary care groups
- clear incentives for all members of the local NHS to improve performance and efficiency
- a national schedule of reference costs, and NHS trusts to publish and benchmark their costs
- clear sanctions when performance and efficiency are not up to standard
- phasing out of extra-contractual referrals, cost per case and short-term contracts.

The NHS in Scotland

The NHS in Scotland has around 132 000 staff, including more than 63 000 nurses, midwives and health visitors, and over 8500 doctors. There are also more than 7000 family practitioners, including doctors, dentists, opticians and community pharmacists providing a range of services within the NHS in return for various fees and allowances. The Scottish Executive Health Department leads the central management of the NHS, heading a Management Executive which oversees the work of 15 area health boards that are responsible for planning health services for people in their area, and 28 self-governing NHS trusts which are responsible for providing services to patients and the community.

Since power was devolved to the Scottish Parliament in 1999, Edinburgh has had primary and secondary legislative powers over health issues. This means that the Scottish Parliament can pass its own laws on a wide range of health topics, but is only able to vary others. Areas which have remained within the control of the English Department of Health include abortion, embryology, surrogacy, genetic fertilisation and medicine safety.

The NHS in Wales

The National Assembly for Wales is responsible for policy direction and for allocating funds to the NHS in Wales. Following the establishment of the National Assembly for Wales, the vast majority of the health responsibilities of the Welsh Office passed to the National Assembly.

The Assembly allocates funds annually to each of the five regional health authorities, which are as follows:

- Bro Taf Health Authority
- Dyfed Powys Health Authority
- Gwent Health Authority
- Iechyd Morgannwg Health Authority
- North Wales Health Authority.

The health authorities buy health services from professionals in primary care, such as family doctors, dentists and opticians, and from the NHS trusts that provide secondary and community care.

As part of the major reform of the NHS, local health groups (LHGs) have been established within each area to provide a local focus for the development and improvement of health services. They will make a major contribution in the following three main areas:

- the development of health improvement programmes (HImPs)
- the development of clinical governance to improve the quality of primary care
- informing and developing the commissioning of hospital and community health services.

Local health groups are committees of the health authorities – the Welsh equivalent of English primary care groups. There are 22 LHGs responsible for commissioning in Wales. These groups were formed in April 1999 and are compulsory for GPs, with each group having a governing body that reflects the range of health professional interests within the locality.

There are also 22 community health councils in Wales, one in each local authority area. They represent issues on behalf of the public.

The NHS in Northern Ireland

The NHS in Northern Ireland is the responsibility of the Secretary of State. In Northern Ireland, personal social services are integrated with health services under the administration of the Department of Health and Social Services. Health services in Northern Ireland are managed by the Health and Social Services Executive (HSSE), which is led by a chief executive supported by six directors.

There are four health and social services boards in Northern Ireland, which function in a similar manner to health authorities in England. They are responsible for identifying and meeting the health and social care needs of their local populations. To meet those identified needs, they contract with service providers, including the health and social services trusts and others in both the private and voluntary sectors.

Since devolution, the emphasis on primary care has increased – more services are delivered through the community rather than through hospital services – with the establishment of primary care groups and trusts. As in other parts of the UK, patient needs are central to the overall health programme.

The impact of devolution appears to be leading to different approaches to the NHS in England, Scotland, Wales and Northern Ireland.

Our Healthier Nation: improving health

The White Paper, *Saving Lives: Our Healthier Nation,* was published in July 1999. The document proposed a new 'contract for health with the people of England', promising to unite the nation in a drive against poor health. The new strategy was designed to replace *The Health of the Nation*, and in place of the 27 target areas of that initiative, four key targets are incorporated in three key aims.

The key aims are as follows:

- to increase the length of our lives

- to increase the number of years we spend living life to the full

- to increase the opportunities for a healthier and longer life for the many and not just for the few.

The four national targets are as follows:

- *heart disease and stroke* – to reduce the death rate from heart disease and stroke in people under 75 years of age by at least two-fifths by 2010

- *accidents* – to reduce the rate of occurrence of major accidents to children and adults by one-fifth by 2010, and to reduce serious injury by one-tenth
- *cancer* – to reduce the death rate from all cancers among people under 65 years of age by 2010 by at least one-fifth
- *mental health* – to reduce the death rate from suicide and undetermined injury by one-fifth by 2019.

Health authorities have important leadership roles in the implementation of *Our Healthier Nation*, and will lead local alliances to develop health improvement programmes.

Health Development Agency (HDA)

The HDA is a special health authority that aims to improve the health of people in England, and in particular to reduce inequalities in health between those who are well off and those who are on low incomes or reliant on state benefits. The HDA came into force in April 2000. The establishment of the HDA was announced in the White Paper, *Saving Lives: Our Healthier Nation*, in the summer of 1999. The White Paper aims to improve the health of everyone, particularly those who are worst off, taking into account the social, economic and environmental factors that affect health. The HDA's role in achieving this aim is to:

- gather evidence of what works
- advise on good practice
- support all those who are working to improve the public's health.

Health Promotion in England (HPE)

HPE was established in April 2000 following the closure of the Health Education Authority. It develops and delivers public education campaigns and promotes healthy living by focusing in particular on the following:

- alcohol
- children and families
- drugs
- immunisation
- older people
- sexual health.

It works in partnership with national and local organisations (both statutory and voluntary), to provide support to health and other professionals at local and community level. It is part of the NHS and works under contract to the Department of Health and the Department of Trade and Industry.

The NHS Plan

This is a plan for investment in the NHS with a sustained increase in funding. It is a plan for reform, with far-reaching changes across the NHS. The purpose and vision of the NHS Plan is to give the people of the UK a health service for the twenty-first century, and a health service designed around the patient. The NHS has delivered major improvements in health, but it falls short of the standards that patients expect and staff want to provide. Public consultation for the plan showed that the public wanted to see the following changes:

- more and better paid staff using new ways of working

- reduced waiting-times, and high-quality care centred on patients

- improvements in local hospitals and surgeries.

In part the NHS is failing to deliver because over the years it has been underfunded. In particular there have been too few doctors, nurses and other key staff to carry out all of the treatments required. However, there have been other underlying problems as well. The NHS is a 1940s system operating in a twenty-first century world, with:

- lack of national standards

- old-fashioned demarcations between staff and barriers between services

- a lack of clear incentives and levers to improve performance

- over-centralisation and disempowered patients.

These systematic problems, which date from 1948 when the NHS was formed, are tackled by the NHS Plan. It has examined other forms of funding healthcare and found them wanting. The systems used by other countries do not provide a route to better healthcare. The principles of the NHS are solid, but its practices need to change.

The March 2000 Budget settlement means that the NHS will grow by half in cash terms and by one-third in real terms in just five years. This is funding extra investment in the following NHS facilities:

- 7000 extra beds in hospitals and intermediate care

- over 100 new hospitals by the year 2010 and 900 new one-stop primary care centres

- 3000 GP premises modernised and 250 new scanners

- clean wards overseen by modern matrons, and better hospital food

- modern IT systems in every hospital and GP surgery.

It is also funding investment in staff as follows:

- 7500 more consultants and 2000 more GPs

- 20 000 extra nurses and 6500 extra therapists

- 1000 more medical school places

- childcare support for NHS staff, with 1000 on-site nurseries.

However, investment is being accompanied by reform. The NHS is being redesigned around the needs of the patient. Local hospitals cannot be run from Whitehall. There is a new relationship between the Department of Health and the NHS to enshrine the trust that patients have in frontline staff. A new system of earned autonomy is devolving power from the centre to the local health service as modernisation takes hold.

The Department of Health now sets national standards that are matched by regular inspection of all local health bodies by the Commission for Health Improvement. A more streamlined centre has included the merging of the posts of Permanent Secretary and Chief Executive, creating one post. Nigel Crisp was appointed to this post in the autumn of 2001.

The National Institute for Clinical Excellence was established to ensure that availability of cost-effective drugs such as those for cancer is not dependent on where one lives. In addition, a Modernisation Agency has been set up to spread best practice.

Local NHS organisations that perform well for patients will be given more freedom to run their own affairs. There is a £500 million performance fund. However, the Government will intervene more rapidly in those parts of the NHS that fail their patients.

For the first time, social services and the NHS have come together with new agreements to pool resources. There will be new care trusts to commission health and social care in a single organisation. This will help to prevent patients – particularly old people – falling into the gap between the two services, or being left in hospital when they could be safely living in their own home.

For the first time there will be modern contracts for both GPs and hospital doctors. NHS doctors work hard for the NHS. However, the contracts under which they work are outdated. There will be a large extension of quality-based contracts for GPs in general, and for single-handed practices in particular. The number of consultants entitled to additional discretionary payments will rise from half to two-thirds, but in return they will be expected to increase their productivity while working for the NHS. Newly qualified consultants will not be able to undertake private work for perhaps as long as seven years.

For the first time nurses and other staff, not just in some places but everywhere, will have a greater opportunity to extend their roles. By 2004, over half of them will be able to prescribe medicines. In total, £280 million is being set aside over the next three years to develop the skills of staff. All support staff will have an Individual Learning Account worth £150 per year. The number of nurse consultants will increase to 1000, and a new role of consultant therapist will be introduced. A new Leadership Centre will be set up to develop a new generation of managerial and clinical leaders, including modern matrons with authority to get the basics right on the ward.

For the first time, patients will have a real say in the NHS. They will have new powers and more influence over the way in which the NHS works, including the following:

- letters about an individual patient's care will be copied to the patient

- better information will help patients to choose a GP

- patient advocates and advisers will be set up in every hospital

- there will be proper redress when operations are cancelled on the day on which they are due to take place

- there will be patients' surveys and forums to help services to become more patient centred.

For the first time there will be a concordat with private providers of healthcare to enable the NHS to make better use of facilities in private hospitals – where this provides value for money and maintains standards of patient care. NHS care will remain free at the point of delivery – regardless of who provides it.

These far-reaching reforms to the service will result in direct improvements for patients. For example, patients will see waiting-times for treatment cut as extra staff are recruited.

- By 2004, patients will be able to have a GP appointment within 48 hours and there will be up to 1000 specialist GPs taking referrals from fellow GPs.

- Long waits in accident and emergency departments will be ended.

- By the end of 2005, the maximum waiting-time for an outpatient appointment will be three months, and for inpatients it will be six months.

The treatment of cancer, heart disease and mental health – the conditions that kill and affect most people – will improve with:

- a large expansion in cancer-screening programmes
- an end to the postcode lottery with regard to the prescribing of anti-cancer drugs
- rapid access to chest pain clinics across the country by the year 2003
- shorter waiting-times for heart operations
- 335 mental health teams to provide an immediate response to crises.

Older people use the NHS more than any other group. The NHS Plan will provide them with both better and new services, including the following:

- national standards for caring for older people to ensure that ageism is not tolerated
- breast screening to cover all women aged 65 to 70 years
- personal care plans for elderly people and their carers
- nursing care in nursing homes to become free
- by 2004, a £9 million package of new intermediate care services to allow older people to live more independent lives.

The NHS plan will bring health improvements across the board for patients, but for the first time there will also be a national inequalities target. To help to achieve this, we will:

- increase and improve primary care in deprived areas
- introduce screening programmes for women and children
- step up smoking cessation services
- improve the diet of young children by making fruit freely available for 4 to 6-year-olds in schools.

The NHS Plan will require investment and reforms to make it work. However, the funding is there to support change and is backed by the key organisations in the NHS. There is a new national alliance behind a reformed patient-centred NHS. These are the most fundamental and far-reaching reforms the NHS has seen since 1948.

Summary

1988
January	Ministerial Review of the NHS.
July	Department of Health created following the splitting up of the Department of Health and Social Security. Kenneth Clarke appointed as Secretary of State for Health.

1989
January	*Working for Patients* is published.
November	*NHS and Community Care Bill* is published.

1990
June	*NHS and Community Care Bill* receives Royal Assent.

1991
April	NHS reforms come into operation. The first wave of 57 NHS trusts and 306 GP fundholders is established in England.
October	The *Patient's Charter* is published.

1992
April	The second wave of 99 NHS trusts and 288 GP fundholders is established in England.
July	White Paper on *The Health of the Nation* is published.
October	Report of the *Tomlinson Inquiry* is published.

1993
February	The Government publishes its response to the *Tomlinson Inquiry*, entitled *Making London Better*. A review of functions and manpower in the NHS is announced.
April	The third wave of 136 NHS trusts and over 600 GP fundholders is established in England.
July	The functions and manpower review reports to ministers.
October	*Managing the New NHS* is published in response to review. This included the proposed abolition of regional health authorities, the merger of district health authorities and family health services authorities, and a streamlining of the NHS management executive.

1994
April	The fourth wave of 140 NHS trusts and 800 GP fundholders is established in England. The NHS management executive is renamed the NHS Executive and establishes eight regional offices. The number of regional health authorities is reduced from 14 to 8.
June	NHS performances tables published for the first time.
October	*Developing NHS Purchasing and GP Fundholding* is published.

1995
January	An updated *Patient's Charter* is published.

April	The fifth wave of 21 NHS trusts and 560 GP fundholders is established in England. An accountability framework for fundholders is introduced.
June	*Health Authorities Bill* receives Royal Assent.
November	Plans to use a private finance initiative to build a new NHS hospital are announced.

1996

April	Regional health authorities are abolished and their functions are taken over by NHS Executive regional offices. District health authorities and family health services authorities are replaced by unitary health authorities. The sixth wave of 1200 GP fundholders is established in England. Around 50 total purchasing projects go live.
June	Consultation paper, *Primary Care: The Future* is published.
October	White Paper on primary care, *Choice and Opportunity*, is published. Reports of NHS funding problems.
November	White Paper on the future of the NHS, *The National Health Service. A Service with Ambitions*, is published. *The NHS (Primary Care) Bill* is published. Additional resources for the NHS are announced.
December	Second White Paper on primary care, *Primary Care: Delivering the Future*, is published.

1997

May	A Labour Government is elected and Frank Dobson is appointed Secretary of State for Health.
December	White Paper, *The New NHS: Modern, Dependable*, is published. White Paper on the future of the NHS in Scotland, *Designed to Care*, is published.

1998

April	First-wave health action zones (HAZs) established. First wave of newly merged trusts is announced.

1999

June	Health Act received Royal Assent and came into force in April 2000. The new NHS reforms, which included quality of care in NHS trusts and responsibility of partnership between the NHS and local authorities.
July	Public health White Paper, *Saving Lives: Our Healthier Nation*, is published.

2000

July	The NHS Plan – *A Plan for Investment, a Plan for Reform*, is published.

2

Patient (customer) care

The medical receptionist and secretary

Medical secretaries and receptionists are important and sometimes undervalued members of the healthcare team. Usually they are the first point of contact that the patient has with a medical practice or a hospital department, clinic or ward. The receptionist's attitude, empathy and efficiency are able either to enhance or to damage their image. A good receptionist can facilitate the way in which a patient accesses the system of medical care, and should do all that is possible to make the patient feel welcome and comfortable, and to ease their access to medical help and care.

The first impression the patient has of the surgery or hospital department is usually of the reception area and the reception staff. Remember that the receptionist is the 'shop window' and the way in which patients feel as they sit in the waiting-area will largely depend on how the receptionist has reacted to and greeted them. It is the receptionist's role to allay patients' fears and worries and help them to feel 'comfortable' whilst they wait. A courteous, friendly manner, accompanied by a smile and an understanding of the situation can work wonders even with the most difficult patients. The secretary, too, often has to reassure anxious patients and their relatives, and should adopt a similar approach.

Everyone, whether they be patients, secretaries, receptionists, doctors or other members of the healthcare team, has feelings. If you have personal problems it is difficult not to let your emotions affect the way in which you respond and interact with patients and colleagues. It is important to be aware of this and develop the ability to overcome your feelings. Your attitude will influence the attitude of the person you are dealing with. Remember that patients have personal problems, too, and are often anxious or frightened, so your empathy with their feelings will do a lot to improve your own attitude.

Box 2.1

How do you welcome patients?

Do you welcome them all in the same way?

Why do you treat people differently?

Why are some patients 'difficult' when they attend a hospital or GP surgery?

What are patients' expectations?

Have you experienced feelings of fear?

How do you react when you are frightened or worried?

How would you like to be treated?

Putting patients first

What is customer care?

Customer care means:

- giving the right impression
- meeting customers' expectations
- exceeding customers' expectations
- listening to customers
- having customer-friendly systems
- being totally professional
- putting customers first
- being totally customer oriented
- having the right attitude
- treating others as you would wish to be treated
- maintaining consistently high standards of service.

Remember that the NHS is a very large business organisation and the customers are your business.

Customer care is not:

- a quick fix
- the flavour of the month
- a campaign which runs for three months and then stops
- just something for the receptionists
- something which brings instant results
- something which starts *after* the patient has reported to the receptionist.

What does the customer expect of us?

Customers have a variety of expectations about the following:

- the product and service
- staff
- the organisation – hospital or GP surgery.

These expectations will include the following:

- welcoming, pleasant, smiling receptionists
- a concern for their needs
- interest and recognition
- value for money
- adequate information
- good support services
- satisfaction of their needs
- quality service.

Every patient/customer matters and deserves the best that you and your practice, hospital or clinic can offer.

Creating the right impression

Box 2.2 Some do's and don'ts for creating the right impression

DO	DON'T
Greet the patient pleasantly	Be rude
Make eye contact	
Use names	Be distant, or call everyone 'dear' or 'love'
Give your full attention	Be bored
	Talk to colleagues when patients need attention
Show respect for the patient	Criticise other members of the healthcare team
Be helpful	Be unco-operative
Be confident	
Be positive	
Be efficient	
Be caring	
SMILE	

What improvements can be made?

By you?

By other members of the team?

YOU NEVER GET A SECOND CHANCE TO MAKE A FIRST IMPRESSION!

A number of factors help to create the right or wrong impression, including the following:

- layout
- space

- signs
- noise
- clutter/rubbish
- staff appearance
- staff behaviour
- facial expression
- tone of voice
- posture.

How to discover the customer's needs

Try to pick up any clues from what is said by the caller, and listen to the 'hidden' message. Do not jump to conclusions about the customer's needs – they are not always clearly expressed.

Follow up and probe by asking questions. Use 'open' questions, starting with the following.

- How?
- Why?
- What?
- When?

However, do not interrogate the customer.

Actively listen in order to discover the customer's needs

- Do not make hasty judgements.
- Do not let personal feelings or prejudices prevent you from listening to what is being said.
- Do not interrupt, even if you feel that you can guess the end of the sentence or remark.
- Do not forget to show that you are listening.
- Do not be distracted.

Body language or non-verbal communication (NVC)

Body language is an important factor in customer care. Remember that it may reflect what you are really thinking! Body language should reinforce the spoken word. When it is contradictory, the customer may well believe the body language and not what is being said.

Important aspects of body language include the following.

- *Facial expressions and head position* – the face is mobile and can register a huge range of expressions. The expression on your face when you welcome the customer will affect their impression of you. Your head position is also important. Tilting your head to one side indicates interest in the other person.

- *Posture* – the way in which you hold your body is important. Observe people in your place of work and you will be surprised at the information you can obtain from their posture. Posture gives an indication of the level of interest in the customer. For example, leaning slightly towards the customer suggests interest and concern, leaning away with the arms folded indicates lack of interest or even boredom, and standing with the hands on the hips is an aggressive signal.

- *Proximity* – we all need our 'personal space'. and people who get too close to us will often make us feel uncomfortable and threatened. You should be close enough to customers to show interest – approximately three to four feet away is usually the best distance.

- *Eye contact and gaze* – looking someone in the eye is generally felt to be a positive signal. Look directly at the customer, albeit briefly, when making the initial welcome. Not looking at them may indicate an attitude of not caring. However, some people avoid eye contact for reasons of shyness or because of cultural tradition. Your eyes probably give the most expressive signal of all. Watch the customer's eyes during a conversation and you will gain feedback as to whether they understand or agree with what you are saying. Aim to meet their gaze for approximately two-thirds of the time.

- *Body contact* – in our society it is not appropriate to touch a complete stranger. In general, the only acceptable form of touching is the handshake when greeting or saying goodbye to a customer.

- *Gestures* – our gestures provide a lot of information (e.g. a nod or a shrug). Negative gestures include finger or foot tapping (impatience or aggression) and yawning (boredom).

- *Tone of voice* – we all convey a great deal of information to people not by what we are saying, but by the tone of our voice. You may use welcoming words, but if you sound disinterested or angry you may cause the patient distress. Always ensure that your tone is as friendly as the actual words spoken.

A good technique is to mirror the customer's body language. Customer care and use of the telephone will be dealt with in Chapter 3.

Complaints within the health service

In recent years there has been increasing public awareness about quality of service. People have higher expectations of the service that they receive. It used to be the case that people only complained if the quality of the goods that they bought was substandard, but nowadays people are equally concerned about how they are treated when they are buying their goods.

This also applies to the health service. People expect to receive a high standard of care and service. If they do not do so, they are becoming more forthright about complaining.

Complaints are taken very seriously in the health service today. In order to develop and maintain a high standard of service we need to know when things go wrong. We need to know what has happened so that it can be avoided in future, and so that action is taken to prevent it from happening again.

We also need to respond to our customers, the patients. If they do not receive the service that they expect, they need to know that they can complain and that their complaint will be investigated. They need to know that their complaint will be taken seriously and that they will receive an explanation and apology, if appropriate.

Moreover, quality standards are written into the contracts between purchasers and provider units. Complaints as an indicator of quality are monitored scrupulously by the purchasers. If a provider unit's services fall continually below the required standard, it is possible that their contract may not be renewed, thus threatening that hospital's very existence. GP fundholders are also unlikely to refer patients to hospitals where there is a high level of complaints about which no action is taken.

Patients have the right to have any complaints about NHS services investigated, and to receive a full written reply. In 1993 the Wilson Committee looked into the existing complaints procedure and found that it had become slow, cumbersome and difficult to access. As a result of the Committee's report, the following set of principles was agreed which should underpin any effective complaints procedure:

- responsiveness

- quality enhancement

- cost-effectiveness

- accessibility

- impartiality

- simplicity

- speed

- confidentiality

- accountability.

These principles provide the foundation for the NHS complaints procedures that were introduced in April 1996. The procedure aims to provide a fair, simple and open system which is easy to access and enables lessons on quality to be extracted and used to improve services for patients. The primary aim is to resolve complaints and satisfy the concerns of the complainant through early, local resolution.

Why do patients complain?

Patients complain about a wide variety of different issues, such as the following:

- postponement of an appointment

- waiting-times for a first outpatient appointment or to see the doctor in the clinic or surgery

- cancellation of an appointment or admission to hospital

- time on the waiting-list

- cancellation or postponement of surgical procedures

- lack of information

- not being kept informed of treatments

- staff behaviour and attitudes

- food

- a doctor not visiting the patient at home

- cleanliness and building debris

- missing medical records, X-rays and test results

- missing property.

The person nominated by the practice or NHS trust to be responsible for dealing with complaints should give information about the procedure to the person who is complaining. This will include, where appropriate:

- how the complaint will be dealt with

- the purpose of the procedure

- the anticipated timetable

- the rules of confidentiality

- the availability of help from the local community health council

- possible outcomes of the procedure, so that the person complaining may have realistic expectations

- the availability of conciliation services through the health authority or health board

- how to pursue a complaint with the health authority if the person who is complaining is not satisfied with the practice-based investigation

- the time limits for making complaints:

  – within six months of the date of the incident that caused the problem
  or
  – within six months of the date of discovering the problem, provided that this is within 12 months of the incident.

Patients have the right to a full and prompt written reply from the Chief Executive to any written complaint against a trust or health authority. The NHS tries to provide this within four weeks of receiving any complaint. Where there are good reasons why this cannot be achieved, patients must be kept informed of progress.

The complaints procedure

The aim of the system is to try to resolve most complaints close to the cause of patients' complaints, be that a doctor, nurse, receptionist, secretary or practice manager. In many cases it should be possible to resolve the problem straight away. This procedure is part of the local resolution mechanism for settling complaints in the NHS; health authorities and health boards can also contribute to the local resolution process through the provision of conciliation services.

If patients feel that they have a reason to complain, they can do so directly to the medical practice or NHS trust concerned. However, health authorities or health boards have complaints managers who may be contacted by patients if they prefer to talk to someone who is not directly involved in their healthcare.

The complaints procedure is currently under review, with no changes expected in the foreseeable future. However, it is anticipated that a new procedure will be introduced in keeping with the recent changes and mergers in the health service.

Complaints procedures in general medical practice

The terms of service of all family health practitioners have been amended to reflect these procedures. All practitioners are required to:

- have a practice-based system for handling complaints, which must comply with the national criteria
- co-operate with their health authority complaints procedures, including independent review, if a complaint proceeds beyond the practice-based system.

National criteria for the NHS complaints procedure are as follows.

- Complaints should be acknowledged within two working days.
- An explanation should be provided within ten working days.
- Practices must publicise their complaints procedure.
- Written information on how to make a complaint must be available and include details of how to complain to a health authority or health board.
- Practices must nominate one person to be responsible for administering the complaints procedure.

Health authority and health board procedure

Health authority procedures are known as Independent Review. In all health authorities a senior member of staff is responsible for managing complaints. He or she works closely with a convenor, who will be a non-executive director of the health authority or a person specifically charged by the board of the trust/health authority to act in this role, and who has responsibility for looking at complaints and deciding whether to agree a request for an Independent Review. The convenor will have access to independent medical advice from a doctor nominated by the Local Medical Committee (LMC). Health authority action must be flexible and does not, as with previous service committee procedures, need to follow strict procedures. The role of the convenor is to:

- refer the complaint back to the practice if it appears that the practice-based procedure has not been exhausted
- arrange conciliation where it appears that this might be helpful. Health authorities have to ensure that conciliation services are available to both parties

COMPLAINT TO CONVENOR

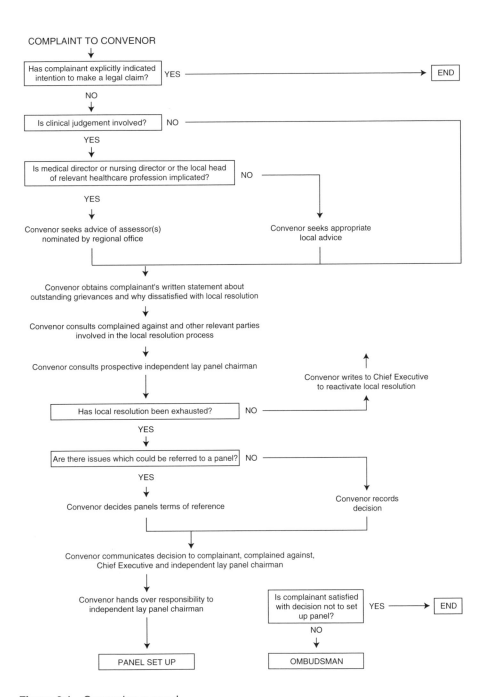

Figure 2.1 Convening a panel.

- set up an independent review panel to investigate the complaint
- take no further action if it is clear that everything that could be done has been done
- advise the complainant of his or her right to approach the Ombudsman.

The Ombudsman

Most complaints should be resolved through one of the procedures. However, if a complainant remains dissatisfied, he or she is able to go to the Health Service Commissioner (Ombudsman), although further consideration is not an automatic right, and the Ombudsman will decide on the merits of each case before embarking on a full investigation.

Receptionists and secretaries are advised to ask their managers for a copy of the complaints procedure used in their healthcare organisation, and for any points about which they are unsure to be explained.

Having a standard procedure also ensures clear communication. In fact, lack of communication is the root cause of many of the complaints that are made in hospitals. A complaint about a relatively minor matter can become quite serious if it is not taken seriously in the first place. Thus having a complaints procedure is better both for patients and for staff. It ensures that complaints are taken seriously, and that everyone involved has an opportunity to express their opinion. It encourages clear communication, and by doing so may reduce complaints in the long term. It can also help to improve the hospital's public image. More importantly, the major benefit of having a procedure is to ensure that the quality of service can be monitored, thus helping to maintain and develop high standards of care. A standardised procedure ensures that the charter standard requirement for a full investigation and written response to all complaints from the Chief Executive is met.

How to meet the Wilson Report requirements

- *Accessibility*: Promote the system with a patient information leaflet and poster, making it clear exactly who patients should approach.
- *Confidentiality*: Agree procedures (e.g. if a third party is involved, give no information without the patient's consent).
- *Impartiality*: Keep all complaints records and file them separately from the patient's medical records.

- *Responsiveness*: Keep patients informed at each stage about how long the complaint will take to resolve. Make them aware of the procedures they can follow if they are dissatisfied.
- *Simplicity*: Keep the procedure and patient information leaflets as simple as possible.
- *Speed*: Encourage complaints to be made quickly and handled as speedily as possible within the stated time-scale. Delays can cause problems to escalate.

Taking customer complaints seriously

All complaints must be taken seriously. If a customer complains, this provides an opportunity to put things right. All complaints should be:

- logged
- passed to the appropriate manager
- acted upon.

Complaints should be dealt with immediately, and the customer should know the outcome as soon as possible. Remember that a complaint is any situation in which the customer is not satisfied. If a complaint is handled well, the customer might feel more loyalty than before.

Box 2.3 Do's and don'ts of complaints

DO	DON'T
Obtain all of the facts	Interrupt
Listen to what the customer has to say	Argue
	Justify
Apologise on behalf of the organisation without making excuses	Make excuses
Show concern	
Tell the customer what will be done	

Patients expect:

- an apology, if appropriate
- a clear explanation
- assurance that action will be taken to prevent a recurrence.

The future – what improvements can be expected?

To avoid things going wrong in the first place, patients and the public will be involved in shaping local services. Depending on legislation, from 2002 the following will apply.

- All NHS organisations will have to ask patients and carers for their views on the services they have received and publish in a patient prospectus what action will be taken as a result. This will be linked to financial rewards to improve standards, and will also include local information on services available (e.g. local voluntary organisations).

- A patient advocacy and liaison service (PALS) will be available in all NHS and primary care trusts to help to resolve problems straight away.

- An independent statutory patients' forum will be set up in every trust (and will for the first time elect a patient to the trust board) so that patients can have their say.

- Each health authority area will have to set up an independent local advisory forum chosen from residents of the area, to provide a sounding board when deciding on local health priorities and policies.

- Health services will be scrutinised by local authorities which have been elected democratically.

- In particular, your local council will scrutinise all major changes to local health services. If the committee involved is not satisfied that the planned changes are in the best interests of the local population, or that there has been enough consultation, they can refer the decision to the newly formed independent Reconfiguration Panel (which will include patient representative members). They will then consider the 'evidence' and give independent advice and recommendations on the decision.

At the moment, the Government is evaluating the complaints procedure. The Government will act on the outcome of this evaluation and reform the complaints procedure to make it more independent and meet patients' needs.

The NHS Plan has introduced new ways to strengthen the complaints and redress procedures when things go wrong.

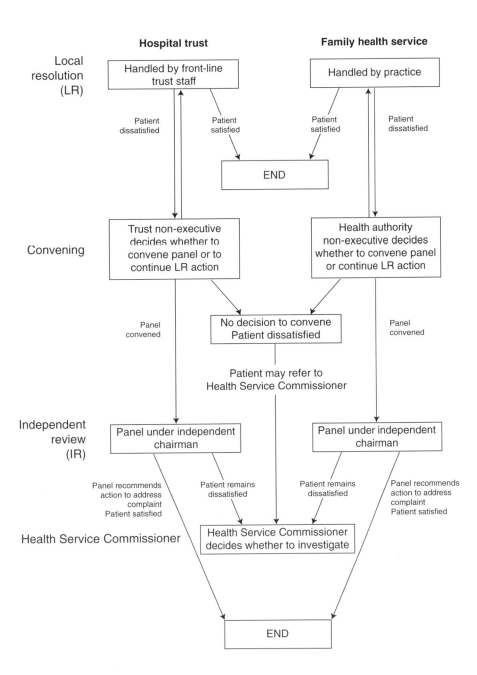

Figure 2.2   Complaints procedure.

Final impressions

The patient must go away feeling satisfied with the level of service you have given. They should feel that you:

- have been willing to help
- have gone to some trouble
- are more co-operative than others.

This will give a good impression of:

- you
- your skills as a secretary or receptionist
- your medical practice or your hospital.

Don't take customers (i.e. patients) for granted.

Summary

Customer care means that you as a medical secretary or receptionist should ensure:

- that your customers are, and feel, welcome (e.g. the way in which you greet them when they arrive will show them whether you care)
- that you show concern for the customer's needs (e.g. by the way in which you listen when they are asking a question or explaining something)
- that you are interested, friendly and pleasant (e.g. by being courteous at all times)
- that you know what you are talking about (e.g. the services that your hospital, practice or clinic offers)
- that the services are the best possible
- that you recognise each customer as an individual person.

The medical secretary and receptionist and customer care

An experienced receptionist's or secretary's responsibility can be boundless and very fulfilling. They are able to assist and understand patients' medical conditions and help accordingly. They may arrange for a wheelchair, a porter or generally provide assistance. They will notice if a patient appears to be distressed and point this out to a nurse or doctor if they consider it necessary. On a practical level, they will keep the reception area generally tidy. For example, magazines will be up to date and in good condition, toys for children will not become a hazard to waiting patients but are kept in a special play area, and plants and flowers will be fresh and watered when necessary. In a private hospital or practice, coffee will no doubt be offered to patients while they wait.

Developing your personal effectiveness

Being assertive

Being assertive means treating other people with respect, asking for what you want and not blaming others for what happens to you. It stems from taking an honest look at strengths and weaknesses and accepting them. Assertive behaviour can include some or many of the mannerisms listed in Box 2.4.

Box 2.4	
Voice	Steady, firm Tone is mid-range, rich and warm Sincere, clear
Speech pattern	Fluent Emphasises key words Steady, even pace Moderate speed
Facial expression	Responsive, matching the feelings expressed Open Steady features Attentive Interested
Eye contact	Direct Maintained
Body	Relaxed Open hand movements (inviting to speak) Sits upright or relaxed (not cowering or slouching) Stands with head held up

This type of behaviour makes other people feel good when they talk to you because you value them and accept their behaviour, and you are not crushed or threatened by rejection because you do not depend on others for approval.

Managing time

To be effective at work, good time management is essential. Box 2.5 identifies some of the problems of poor management of time, the causes, and some possible solutions.

Box 2.5		
PROBLEM	*CAUSES*	*POSSIBLE SOLUTIONS*
Having too much to do	Unclear priorities	Check goals or tasks clearly with your manager and check priorities. Each day, decide on your priorities and stick to them
	Wanting to be directly involved with everything	Be selective, and delegate if you can
	Unrealistic time estimates	Recognise that everything takes longer than you think – add 20% to your estimates
	Overwhelming pressure and piles of paper	Do not confuse activity with effectiveness – just because you are busy this does not mean that you are working well. Try to get into a fixed daily routine with definite times for jobs such as sorting the post, filing, etc.
Inability to finish things	Lack of deadlines	Always set deadlines
	Lack of respect for your time and interruptions by others	Fix a regular time when you need to be left undisturbed. Arrange to divert telephone calls, and agree to accept colleagues' calls in return. Be sure that you know what you want to achieve so that you can communicate this to others
	Doing too many jobs at once	Do one job at a time. When you start a piece of work, try to finish it if you can.

	You waste time each time you have to go back to it, while you remember where you had got to. Be systematic, as then if you have to leave a job part finished, it will make it easier for you, or indeed anyone else, to pick it up again
Wasting time	Handle telephone calls promptly and write messages down immediately. When you make calls, plan what you are going to say beforehand and have all the necessary information to hand
Lack of overview and perspective	Know your priorities. Use your diary. Try to transfer responsibility for some of your work when taking on new jobs. Fix a specific time for any major jobs which should not be interrupted
	Impose deadlines on yourself and tell others about them

Looking after yourself

There is greater pressure than ever before on healthcare staff to work to maintain and improve the health of the community that they serve. A variety of initiatives come immediately to mind – antenatal and postnatal care, family planning, child development and immunisation clinics, screening (well-man, well-woman, elderly), health promotion programmes for specific conditions (e.g. diabetes, hypertension, asthma), healthy eating and anti-smoking advice, and health education literature and posters.

In a more general sense, everyone knows in theory at least that they should take certain basic sensible steps to maintain a healthy lifestyle, but for this to become a reality each individual has to understand how they can help themselves to avoid health problems. In doing this, they will also be contributing to their own personal effectiveness both at work and at home.

Whether you are a doctor, a receptionist, a secretary or a nurse, the message is clear. You will do no one a good service if you do not build in time for looking after yourself.

Paying attention to your own health means taking a hard look at those factors which are known to contribute to poor health, including smoking, drinking to excess and being overweight, and making a conscious effort to take exercise, eat healthily and take advantage of all of the health-screening checks that are available.

Handling stress at work

Most people when discussing their jobs would refer at some point to the amount of pressure that they are under at work. Hopefully this will not be a constant problem, and in fact many people claim to work better when under slight pressure. The problems arise when the pressure becomes too great or continues for a long time.

An awareness of the difference between pressure and stress is important. Generally speaking, stress does not produce a positive or energetic response, but is reflected by panic reactions, irritability, an inability to relax and difficulty with relationships. It is also well known and well established that stress can lead to a variety of medical problems.

Stress at work may have a number of causes. The job may require a great deal of effort, or rapid decision making, or its requirements may be ambiguous and therefore lead to competing demands. Unsatisfactory working conditions, inconsiderate bosses or supervisors, shift work and so on can all put pressure on an individual's ability to cope.

Stress is a fact of life and cannot be eliminated. Indeed, most people would quickly become bored if too few demands were placed on them. The key issue is therefore that of coping – that is, the response made by an individual who encounters a situation with a potentially harmful outcome. Most people employ an enormous number of ways of coping with diverse demands, and often different combinations of different types. In general terms there are two major functions of coping. One is to alter the situation causing stress, and the other is to deal with the emotion that the stress engenders. The extent to which an individual is able to deal with these two aspects depends on a variety of circumstances. However, the fact that they both have an impact in varying degrees can help both in understanding situations better and in developing coping strategies.

Flexibility is important. It is more effective to use a variety of coping skills than to use one specific response. It is therefore necessary to be cautious when taking on board any fixed ideas on how to cope. However, there are some general guidelines which can help one to think through the situation (*see* Box 2.6).

Box 2.6

Know yourself and the way in which you react.

Relax.

Decide what is important.

Look for support from others.

Keep communicating.

Use a step-by-step, problem-solving approach.

Patients' rights and NHS Charter standards

Charter standards were first introduced with the Patient's Charter in 1992 which established certain rights for patients and specific National Charter standards. The Charter set out clear standards of service for patients and basic rights. Those rights for the family doctor service include the following:

- to be registered with a GP

- to change doctors quickly and easily

- to receive emergency care at any time through a family doctor

- to have appropriate drugs and medicines as prescribed

- to be referred to an acceptable consultant when the family doctor considers this is necessary, and to be referred for a second opinion if the patient and their family consider it desirable

- to have access to personal medical records, subject to any limitations by law

- to know that those working for the NHS are under a legal duty to keep the contents of health records confidential

- to choose whether or not to take part in medical research or student training

- to be given detailed information about local family doctor services

- to receive a copy of the doctor's practice leaflet, setting out the services that they provide

- to receive a full and prompt reply to any complaint made about NHS services.

Other elements of the NHS Charter include reducing waiting-times for hospital appointments and operations (which also includes a waiting-time guarantee). Other standards refer to community care services, dental, optician, pharmacy, ambulance and maternity services. The NHS Plan states a commitment that from 2002, if operations are cancelled by the hospital on the day of surgery for non-clinical reasons, the hospital will have to offer another date within the next 28 days. If they cannot do this, they will pay for the patient's treatment at the time and hospital of his or her choice.

The NHS Plan has stated that the current Charter will be replaced. As a result, the Government has published a booklet entitled *Your Guide to the NHS*. This guide helps to explain how changes will affect patients, and how extra resources will produce better services for patients. It sets out what patients can expect from today's NHS and what can be expected in the future. The booklet outlines the NHS Core Principles, which are stated as follows.

Our commitment to you – we want the NHS to be a high-quality health service. These are our aims as set out in the NHS Plan.

- The NHS will provide a universal service for all based on clinical need, not ability to pay.
- The NHS will provide a comprehensive range of services.
- The NHS will shape its services around the needs and preferences of individual patients, their families and their carers.
- The NHS will respond to the different needs of different populations.
- The NHS will work continuously to improve quality services and to minimise errors.
- The NHS will support and value its staff.
- Public funds for healthcare will be devoted solely to NHS patients.
- The NHS will keep people healthy and work to reduce health inequalities.
- The NHS will respect the confidentiality of individual patients and provide open access to information about services, treatment and performance.

This booklet is freely available in GP surgeries, health centres and hospitals. Copies may be obtained by telephoning the Health Literature Line on Freephone 0800 555777. The booklet is available in several languages.

Local charter standards

In addition to the stated National Charter standards, the Government requires health authorities to set clear local standards on areas, including the following:

- waiting-times, including for first outpatient appointments and in other areas as given below

- enabling patients and visitors to find their way around hospitals, through the use of enquiry points and better signposting

- ensuring that staff who deal with patients face to face wear name badges

- nine out of ten patients referred to hospital by GPs or dentists can expect to be given an appointment within 13 weeks, and everyone can expect to be seen within 26 weeks

- the guarantee of a maximum waiting-period of 18 months for hip, knee and cataract operations has been extended to cover all admissions to hospital

- in addition, patients can expect treatment within one year for coronary artery bypass grafts and some associated procedures. (If the consultant considers that the need for treatment is urgent, patients can expect to be seen more quickly.)

Hospitals and trusts are expected to provide enquiry points and clear sign-posting in hospitals, and patients can expect to be cared for in an environment which is clean and safe. Hospitals and trusts are expected to set local standards on:

- waiting-times in accident and emergency departments after the patient's need for treatment has been assessed

- waiting-times for taking patients home after treatment if there is a medical need for NHS transport.

In addition, hospitals and trusts should:

- display information on local standards and whether they are meeting them

- make it clear to patients how they can complain or make comments/ suggestions while they are in hospital

- publish on a regular basis details of the numbers of complaints that they have received and the time taken to deal with them.

Note that expectations are standards of service which the NHS aims to achieve.

Mental health services

A 1997 Department of Health publication clearly stated how the rights and standards in the Patient's Charter apply to individuals using adult mental health services. It gave information about care under the Mental Health Act, and explained how in some circumstances the Mental Health Act overrides certain rights, such as the right to choose whether or not to receive treatment.

The National Service Framework for mental health

The aim of all National Service Frameworks is to improve quality and to reduce unacceptable variations in health and social services for people with certain conditions. The National Service Framework for mental health:

- sets national standards and defines service models for promoting mental health and treating mental illness
- sets time-scales and a specific group of high-level performance targets against which progress will be measured.

Performance targets include the following:

- service users to be given a care plan that is explained by their care co-ordinator
- prescribing of antidepressants and other drugs to be monitored and reviewed within the local clinical audit programme by 2001.

Community care

Local authorities should have a charter covering community services for people with mental health problems who are receiving care in the community.

Access to healthcare

The NHS Plan also commits to improved access to healthcare. Both NHS Direct and NHS walk-in centres provide better access to healthcare.

Consider the ways in which medical secretaries and receptionists ensure that all patients receive the best service and support. This will mean attending to the following:

- the general needs of all patients and visitors

- the special needs of some patients, especially those concerned with mobility, disability, the elderly and ethnic minorities

- patient transport.

Many patients, some of whom will also have special needs, are anxious and uneasy about their visit to the surgery or hospital. The receptionist is usually the first person with whom a patient will communicate, and the special skills, knowledge, understanding and empathy that the receptionist uses when receiving and dealing with the patient are very important.

Patients' general needs

Secretaries and receptionists should be able to answer all queries about the services offered by the practice or hospital department, and to direct patients and give them appropriate information, for example about the following:

- waiting-area

- clinic or surgery times

- relevant consulting-room

- toilet, including disabled facilities

- changing facilities

- refreshment facilities (machines, snack bar, etc.).

Patients' special needs

'Disabled' means being unable to do some of the things that able-bodied people can do. A recent survey shows that approximately 15% of adults have some form of disability.

Disabilities may be present from birth, or they may be the results of accident or disease, which may require a change in lifestyle. However, an ever-increasing group of disabled people are those whose disability develops with age.

The main types of disability are as follows:

- difficulties in mobility

- impaired sight or hearing

- learning difficulties.

People with mobility difficulties may include patients with multiple sclerosis, spina bifida or injury, who are unable to walk and are confined to a wheelchair, or the elderly who walk slowly and awkwardly. People with learning difficulties also include those who have difficulty in reading or writing, which is still common.

Problems may arise when a person with a disability visits the surgery or hospital, and these may be due to the following:

* the premises
* the staff
* the patient.

Premises

Look at your place of work in a detached manner and imagine how it must be for a disabled person. Can a patient in a wheelchair readily gain access to the surgery premises or to your hospital department? Are there steps? Are the doors sufficiently wide for wheelchair access? Where can the wheelchair be placed in the waiting-area? Is there good light at the reception desk to aid lip-reading? Is there an area or room away from the reception desk where confidential matters may be dealt with, or for a private discussion with a deaf person? Are the notices clearly written and easy to read?

Staff

Empathy is the most important quality for any staff dealing with patients, but especially when dealing with disabled patients. Staff should be aware of the disability and anticipate what the difficulties may be. For example, sitting in a waiting-room and worrying that a call may be missed makes a deaf person very anxious. Secretaries and receptionists should be tactful and relate to the patient, help with the difficulties caused by the disability and allow more time to deal with their special needs.

Patients

You will find that the majority of patients with a disability are usually less demanding than many other patients. They try to be as independent as possible, although they are very much aware that special allowances may have to be made because they may be slower, or require things to be written down for them or, if they are in a wheelchair, they may take up more space in the waiting-area.

Secretaries and receptionists should be aware that some patients will try to hide their disability, and you should respect their wishes by offering advice without drawing attention to their problems.

Elderly patients

The medical secretary or receptionist should be aware of the many and diverse problems which may affect an elderly patient's access to healthcare, and try to minimise the effect of some of the following problems which may be encountered:

- impaired hearing

- impaired eyesight

- decreased mobility

- difficulty or inability to cope with new procedures

- reduced energy

- arthritic joints

- fear of being misunderstood

- fear of not understanding instructions

- a desire not to be a nuisance to doctors and staff

- socio-economic problems (e.g. financial problems, loneliness, increasing difficulty in day-to-day living).

Cultural issues and language barriers

Medical secretaries and receptionists should be able to identify an individual patient's ethnic or cultural needs and remember that their manner and the way in which they communicate with patients are important in ensuring that ethnic or cultural requirements are identified and met. Remember that if a patient is discourteous to you, it may be because they have difficulty in expressing themselves, or because they are worried about their medical condition. You should remain professional, polite and calm at all times.

Interpreters

Good communication plays a vital role in the provision of effective healthcare. Many patients, especially in inner-city areas, may have a very limited knowledge of the English language, and an interpreter may have to be used.

An interpreter may be available in some hospitals, or colleagues within the workforce may be able to help. On the other hand, interpreters are available from external sources and receptionists and secretaries should know how to contact them if it is felt that an interpreter may be of significant help in improving communication and understanding.

Patients may be accompanied by a relative or friend who is more fluent in the English language, when attending surgery or a hospital clinic, in order to facilitate communication.

Remember that there are still many people in this country who are illiterate. You should be particularly aware and sensitive when offering your help, as they are often extremely embarrassed about this.

Staff working in general practice will no doubt have a list of interpreting services available locally, or will be able to obtain information from their local authority social services department.

The decision as to which is used will depend on the purpose for which the interpreter's services are required.

External interpreters should be used:

• for formal communications (e.g. interviews, complaints procedures, etc.)

• if requested by the patient, relative or fellow professional involved in the care of the patient

• if professional services are deemed to be necessary to enhance understanding.

Visually impaired people

Guidelines are available from the Royal National Institute for the Blind (RNIB) for the provision of a 'user-friendly' environment for people with poor eyesight. These guidelines give suggestions for improving visibility and for providing tactile and auditory clues.

Visibility

Appropriate lighting is the most important aid to vision. People with visual impairment will need twice the quantity of light that is required by sighted people. As people get older, the need for effective lighting increases. The decor of the surgery or hospital should reflect the needs of people with impaired sight, and the use of contrasting colours will reduce disability. Shiny surfaces create reflection and glare, and if possible their use should be avoided. Obstructions must be kept to a minimum and highlighted. Be aware of potential hazards to the visually impaired, including the following:

• furniture

- planters
- toys left on the floor.

Ideally, all edges to furniture and walls should be rounded to minimise injury in the event of a collision. Signs and notices should be clearly written to be effective.

Any auditory clues that may be used must be direct, useful and readily understood.

Tactile clues and texture contrasts can be underfoot, or at a suitable height for hand/finger touch, enabling the visually impaired person to identify a particular area, etc.

All staff who have contact with visually impaired people can do much to facilitate their access to healthcare.

- Ensure that all instructions are clear and readily understood.
- If necessary, take the person to a seat (they may not be able to see it), and then guide their hand to touch the seat or the back of the chair.
- Take them to the doctor's consulting-room, or to the nurse.
- Arrange help if they need to go from one hospital department to another.
- Help patients with poor eyesight to fill in forms, and if they need to sign their name, place their finger on the place of signature.
- When addressing the patient, use their name, or touch them so that they know you are talking to them and not someone else. When you leave them, don't forget to tell them, so that they do not continue a conversation with someone who is not there.
- Use speech appropriate to people with impaired sight.
- Make sure that they are sitting safely, and that the doctor or nurse can see them.

People with hearing difficulties

Patients who have hearing difficulties or who are totally deaf may wish to communicate in writing, so make sure that you have a supply of pens and paper available. Perhaps some members of staff may be able to use sign language.

If you are dealing with appointments, it is a good idea to make a note in the appointments book of any such patients, so that they are not overlooked when their name is called out and so miss their appointment.

The following points will help you to communicate effectively with people who have hearing difficulties.

Face to face

- Speak up, but do not shout.

- Speak a little more slowly than usual.

- Maintain eye contact.

- Ensure that your face is well lit.

- Make sure that the person can see your face clearly to help lip-reading.

- Do not look away from the person when you are talking to them.

- If you cannot get the message across, write it down.

Telephone

- Speak up, but do not shout.

- Speak more slowly than usual.

- If the patient does not understand you, do not repeatedly use the same words, but instead rephrase what you are saying.

- When giving letters, use letters of the alphabet to clarify ('A' for apple, 'C' for Charlie, etc.).

- When giving numbers, appointment dates, etc., always ask the person to repeat them to ensure that they have understood.

People with learning difficulties

Staff working in both general practice and hospitals will find that they are dealing more and more with people with learning difficulties, who are now living in the community and have the same access to healthcare as anyone else. It is important that they are treated in precisely the same way, but making allowance where necessary to ensure that they get the best out of the health service. Therefore:

- be patient

- do not be intimidated – frustration at being unable to make themselves understood may make people with learning difficulties appear aggressive

- stay calm

- ignore any strange mannerisms and comments

- speak in simple, straightforward language.

Remember that there are still patients who are illiterate and who experience problems in accessing healthcare, perhaps when telephoning for an appointment for pathology or the antenatal clinic, for example. Although they may not be able to read what is written down, they may well be able to name individual letters, so be patient and ask them to give you the letters that form the written word, rather than subjecting them to the embarrassment of admitting to you that they are unable to read.

Children

Many children each day attend their doctor's surgery, the local hospital or community clinic. Everything should be done to provide for children's needs, including the following:

- a play area

- sturdy toys

- colourful books

- a changing area for babies and toddlers.

Again, if possible, chairs and tables in waiting-areas should have rounded corners to prevent serious injury.

Children are often frightened by a surgery or hospital, so staff should be sensitive to the special needs of children and do all that they can to provide a safe, reassuring and friendly environment.

In 1993 the Audit Commission published a report, entitled *Children First*, on the care of sick children. The report examined six principles of care and gave guidance as to how each of these should be adopted.

- *Child and family-centred care*: Hospitals should be sensitive to the special needs of children and their families when in hospital, placing as much emphasis on the care and support of the child (which means the involvement of parents in their care) as on their medical needs. Services also need to be tailored to the wide range of children (from under one year up to 18 years of age).

- *Specially skilled staff*: Children should only be cared for by staff who are specially trained to meet their particular needs.

- *Separate facilities*: Children should only be cared for in facilities which have been designed with their needs in mind. Where separate designed facilities do not exist, children should not be treated in other parts of a hospital.

- *Effective treatments*: Children should only receive treatments which are known to be effective.

- *Appropriate hospitalisation*: Children should only be admitted to hospital when the treatment and care cannot be provided in an alternative environment (e.g. in their home).

- *Strategic commissioning*: Purchasers should be commissioning the types of service which most closely meet children's needs, particularly the development of hospital-at-home services to avoid hospitalisation as far as possible.

The National Association for the Welfare of Children in Hospital (NAWCH) has added to these principles in its Charter for Children in Hospital.

Working people

General practitioners and hospitals alike are becoming aware of the need to improve access to healthcare for working men and women by offering appointments at times that are better suited to their working hours. As a result, surgeries and clinics are offering appointments earlier in the morning, later in the evening, or reserving the first appointments for business people. Similar consideration is being given to mothers with children at school and to the elderly, by offering appointments at appropriate times during the day.

Transport

Patients with their own transport

Many patients will attend both hospital and general practice by car, and although hospitals are now providing more car-parking facilities for all patients, special consideration should be given to the elderly or those with physical difficulties by providing parking facilities as near as possible to the clinic that they are attending.

Similarly, although surgeries may not have the space to provide adequate parking for all patients, special consideration should be given to the elderly and patients with special needs to provide ease of access to healthcare.

Patients using public transport

Receptionists should be able to inform patients about local bus and train services, and to direct them to the appropriate pick-up/drop-off points to enable them to reach their destinations. Information about local taxi services should also be available to patients.

Patients using the ambulance service

Receptionists should be aware of the categories of patients who are eligible for transport by ambulance to and from hospital (walking with assistance, sitting or stretcher cases). Eligibility is assessed by general practitioners or social services, and receptionists will usually be asked by the GP to arrange appropriate transport for the patient's first visit to hospital. Subsequent transport for hospital attendance may be arranged by the hospital receptionist or secretary, but may also be arranged directly by the hospital's ambulance service administrator.

Total quality in medical practice

The phrase 'total quality' is frequently used without any definition of what total quality actually means for the organisation concerned.

NHS trusts, health authorities and GPs are concerned to provide a quality service to their patients (customers), and many of them are committed to a total quality programme. An appropriate definition of total quality in providing health care might be as follows:

> *a cost-effective system for integrating the continuous quality improvement efforts of all involved in healthcare to deliver services which ensure patient (customer) satisfaction.*

Box 2.7

Total quality strives to create a climate for excellence.

Total quality strives to prevent errors rather than to correct them.

Total quality is based on effective and harmonious teamwork with the absolute commitment of all members of the team.

What is a doctor's view of quality?

What is the patient's view?

What is your view?

Patients want easy access to a doctor either in hospital or in general practice. They would prefer to wait in pleasant surroundings and they want as short a waiting-time as possible. They want a reasonable amount of time set aside for their consultation, and they expect receptionists and secretaries to smile, and be sympathetic, and responsive to their needs.

A doctor's perception of quality is probably very different, but they too expect an efficient service from their clerical staff as well as from the medical team in providing patient care.

Receptionists, secretaries, nurses and other members of the healthcare team all have different perceptions of quality. They cannot be expected just to provide an 'excellent' service while auditing themselves. They must be given the opportunity to share in the vision of what the organisation is attempting to achieve. To do the job well, everyone will need guidelines. Clear goals and objectives must be set and regular reviews and training given to help them to create the climate for excellence.

Team members will be encouraged to set their own objectives and to monitor and improve their individual performance. They should be able to make suggestions for improved working methods and to discuss new ideas for improving the service.

Total quality is an extension of customer care, in which every receptionist and secretary working in the field of healthcare plays a vital role.

Audit and quality

Audit in healthcare may be defined as the monitoring and appraisal of performance against predetermined standards and targets in order to provide a quality service and care for the patient.

The NHS Plan: the role of patients

The NHS Plan promises that patients will have considerably more involvement in the NHS than ever before, and that they will have influence at every level. Patients will be expected to have some involvement in various health-related organisations.

Independent local advisory forum

By 2002, each health authority will have to establish an independent local advisory forum, chosen from residents of the area, to provide a sounding board for deciding health priorities and policies. The forum will have a say about the area's health improvement programme which sets out the framework for improving health, reducing inequalities and delivering faster, more responsive services of a consistently high standard.

Local council for independent scrutiny

By 2001, any major planning decisions made by local NHS organisations will also have to be referred to the local council for independent scrutiny. If the committee does not support the proposed changes, it has the power to refer the plans to the national independent Reconfiguration Panel. The panel will advise the Government on whether to approve the proposals. This is the first time that locally elected representatives will have a say in the provision of local health services.

Patient advocacy and liaison services

From 2002, trusts running hospitals, GP practices or front-line community health services would have a patient advocacy and liaison service (PALS).

Patients and carers will be able to turn to PALS whenever they have a problem to resolve or they wish to air concerns about the treatment, care or support that they are receiving.

Rather than just helping patients to complain after the event has occurred, PALS will have direct access to the trust's chief executive and the power to negotiate an immediate solution.

In recent months, a series of meetings has taken place with people who are already involved in representing patients and the public in the NHS to gather views on how to create an advocacy service that can be applied across the NHS. This will help to produce guidelines for trusts on how to set up a PALS.

Patients' forums

By 2001, each trust will also have a patients' forum consisting of patients and representatives from patient and voluntary groups. It will have the power to visit trust facilities to check on standards, including cleanliness and food quality.

The forum will elect one member to be a non-executive director on the trust board, ensuring that patients and their needs are at the very heart of decision making. PALS and forums will also feed patients' complaints back into the system to ensure that the right lessons are learned and steps are taken to ensure that problems are tackled.

From 2003, all hospital, primary care and community trusts will have to ask patients and carers for their views on the services that they have received. In addition, every NHS organisation and care home will have to publish a patient prospectus each year giving an account of the views received from patients and what has been done as a result.

Patient prospectuses

These will set out the range of local services which are available, the ratings that they have received from patients, and the place that they occupy in the national performance tables.

Annual patients' surveys

Patients will be regularly asked for their views on health services through an annual Patients' Survey conducted by all NHS trusts.

Financial rewards will be linked to survey results, so that there is an incentive for NHS organisations to act upon people's views.

Patient groups will be consulted on the issues that should be raised in patient surveys, and surveys will start to take place in 2001 (*see* www.nhs.uk/patientsvoice).

Customer care: involving patients and the public

As a receptionist or secretary you may be involved in using questionnaires or short interview surveys to gather information, views and suggestions from patients and the public to provide an opportunity for them to express their opinions or decisions about healthcare or about local health service provision. Surveys are often designed at different levels:

• for patients and their own healthcare

• for patients and the public about the range of services

• when organising and planning service developments

(*Source*: Chambers R (2000) *Involving Patients and the Public*. Radcliffe Medical Press, Oxford.)

The NHS Executive regards user and public participation as an important priority for all primary care groups, and believes that users of the NHS should have a greater voice and influence.

A national survey of NHS patients that has already been conducted confirms that patients want a fast and convenient health service, which is more in tune with the needs of the modern world. It also shows that people want a certain level of change and modernisation, and the need to shape and deliver its services in the same way.

The NHS Plan aims to restructure the health service from the patient's perspective and to give the patient more information and choice and to protect them from poor-quality service. This reflects the results of the 2000 survey.

NHS Direct and walk-in centres are part of the Government's plan to provide a more patient-focused health service.

Receptionists and secretaries will therefore, from time to time, be asked to assist with medical practice or health department satisfaction surveys or patient surveys, by gathering or collating information. This is all part of the customer care policy of your organisation, which is designed to highlight areas where an improvement in patient service is indicated.

Summary

In this chapter we have looked at the contribution made by both receptionists and secretaries in the health service in their dealings with patients, and their role in creating the first impression that patients have of the healthcare provided in both primary and secondary care.

Quality of healthcare provision and customer care go hand in hand to achieve ever improving standards and patient satisfaction.

3

Communication

Introduction

Communication is the technical term for passing on information. Effective communication occurs when appropriate information is not only passed on, but is seen to be understood and acted upon. Therefore the skills of communication involve the following:

- listening to and understanding what the patient/doctor requires
- conveying appropriate information
- checking that the information has been understood
- checking that a suitable response has been or will be made.

Box 3.1

For the medical receptionist the responsibility of communicating with patients is:

to *listen* first

then to give *appropriate* information

to *check by questioning* that the patient understands

and to *confirm* by observing whether action will be or has been taken whilst *maintaining confidentiality*.

Listening

Listening involves not merely hearing the words that are said, but also hearing what is not said, using intuition, common sense and reading behaviour to obtain the complete picture. On the telephone this is more difficult because body language (*see* Chapter 2) cannot be seen. However, it is important to tune into variations in tone of voice. With patients who are well known this will be an almost automatic process, but with those who are new it is even more important to exercise perception in order to get off to a good start.

The receptionist is the key person in ensuring that information is conveyed between patients, healthcare staff, hospitals, general practices, drug company representatives, pharmacists, suppliers and health authorities/health boards – to name but a few! It is vital that all of the communication skills are used to best effect.

The receptionist needs to be skilled in all forms of communication – verbal, in written form on paper, or by electronic means – but the majority of a receptionist's time will be spent in verbal communication.

Box 3.2

DO	*DON'T*
Speak clearly	Eat or drink while speaking
One thing at a time – give 100% attention to each patient	Do two things at once (e.g. hunt for missing files, or work on the VDU while speaking to someone)
Use words carefully	Use 'slang' or medical jargon to patients
Control conversations with patients – use open and closed questions	Allow the patient to keep you longer than is necessary
Be aware of your own tone of voice	Allow anger or frustration to show in your tone of voice

Use of questions in communicating

Awareness of the use of questions can help the receptionist to draw out patient needs or wrap up an unduly lingering conversation. Although a certain amount of questioning will be done automatically, or according to the practice/hospital policy, when difficulty is encountered, using the right questions will help.

The simplest classification of questions is that they can be open, closed or leading.

* *Open* questions ease the patient into giving the information that is required. For example, 'How can I help you?' encourages the patient to state their need (for an appointment, test result, etc.).

* *Leading* questions encourage the patient to make a decision by stating alternatives from which one needs to be selected. For example, 'Do you want the appointment on Monday or Tuesday?', to which the logical answer is one of the two on offer, or 'You want to give up smoking, don't you?', to which the expected answer is 'Yes'.

* *Closed* questions bring the conversation to a halt. For example, 'Shall I tell the doctor you need to speak to him?', to which the logical answer can only be 'Yes' or 'No'.

Box 3.3

OPEN QUESTIONS begin with the words	*CLOSED QUESTIONS* begin with the words
When . . . .?	Would you . . . .?
How . . . .?	Shall I . . . .?
Who . . . .?	Are you . . . .?
What . . . .?	Do you . . . .?
Where . . . .?	May I . . . .?

Note: This is why 'May I help you?' is a poor way to address someone when you really want to help them, because the instant answer is either 'No', which is difficult for a British person to say outright to someone they do not know, or 'Yes', but this does not help the person to formulate their requirement!

Methods of communication

Communication is the way in which we transmit information, knowledge, thoughts and ideas from one person to another or to a group of people. In any organisation, large or small, communication is important for the business to function effectively.

The four main methods of communication are as follows:

- the spoken word (direct – face to face)

- the written word (e.g. diagrams, posters, notice-boards, etc.)

- the use of telephone systems, including facsimile, answering machines, VDUs, email, etc.

- non-verbal communication (body language) (*see* Chapter 2).

Communication: internal and external

Communication may be either internal or external. The following are examples of written communication.

Written messages

Secretaries and receptionists are always conveying urgent and non-urgent messages from patients or other professionals. It is vital that the messages do not get mislaid and that appropriate action is taken. They should contain the following information:

- the date and time when the message is received

- the name, address and telephone number of the caller

- the name of the intended recipient of the message

- a clearly written and concise message

- the name or initials of the person taking the message.

Memorandum

A memorandum (memo) is an internal written communication which may be used to convey short messages and information either to individuals or to all members of the healthcare team. Your organisation will no doubt use a memorandum form which has several headings.

Notice-boards

Notice-boards can be used to convey information both internally to the organisation and externally to visitors. Notice-boards should be positioned so that they are readily visible and accessible to all who are expected to see the notices displayed. They should be kept up to date, and a member of the team will no doubt have responsibility for this.

White-boards

These are often used in organisations to display information relevant to the day. Hospitals and surgeries may display notices about clinics running late, or health promotion information, etc.

Leaflets and posters

Hospitals and surgeries alike have access to a vast quantity of health promotion material and health messages to patients. Managers will often give receptionists responsibility for displaying leaflets and posters, which should be shown in such a way as to give impact to the intended message.

Protocols and procedures

All healthcare organisations will provide written protocols to communicate to members of the team the procedures for the activities in which staff are involved. Written protocols contain standards of quality, and should be written so that all members of the team involved in the task fully understand the procedures and thus achieve their objectives.

External written communication

Letters remain the most widely used method of written communication. Secretaries will be trained to provide a high standard of letter writing.

Letters are used to communicate with health authorities, NHS trusts, health authorities, health boards, medical professionals and patients. For example, GPs write referral letters to hospital consultants, and hospitals send discharge letters and reports to GPs.

Computers now provide a networking facility linking hospitals, health authorities, laboratories and medical practices.

Report writing

Medical receptionists and secretaries may be asked to investigate a procedure or system that is not running smoothly, or to give an account of an event or incident which has occurred.

Reports are written on a given subject to:

• convey information and ideas

• sometimes convey recommendations.

The features of a good report are that:

• it is easily understood

• it is always clear

• it is as long as it needs to be, but no longer.

A report must be complete and accurate with regard to the information it conveys and, because a decision may be based on the report, it must be correct.

A logical structure for the type of report you may be asked to present would be as follows.

1   Introduction:

• subject heading or title

• terms of reference – what you have been asked to find out

• procedure – how you found this out.

2   Body of report:

• findings – what you have found out.

3   Conclusion:

• conclusions – your conclusion or diagnosis

• recommendations – what you think should be done.

Medical receptionists and secretaries may be asked to type more detailed reports, some of which may require a formal business format. There will no doubt be a 'house-style' which should be used, otherwise reference to a manual of basic secretarial skills will give the necessary guidelines.

Note: A report must be accurate, clear, concise and logically arranged. It should be concise to the extent that there is no 'padding' or irrelevant detail.

Electronic mail

Electronic mail or email has become very much a part of our means of communication, both in our private lives and in the workplace.

It is an important and useful communication tool, as it allows us to communicate information, or to leave messages for our colleagues and professional people countrywide and all over the world, 24 hours a day.

Email allows the speedy and efficient transmission of information, enabling decisions to be reached more quickly and thus contributing to a more effective service.

Telephone skills

Telephone callers only have tone of voice and words to go upon. Any frustrations that are felt at the time of answering the phone will be conveyed to the caller in the tone of voice and intonation of the words.

It is difficult to illustrate this point from the written word. However, consider the common phrase used by many organisations to answer the telephone: 'How can I help you?' This can be said with genuine interest, conveyed by a warmth of tone. Alternatively, it can be said in a robotic tone which makes the caller feel as if they want to leave a message on an answer-machine for someone else to call back later!

Understandably, by 10.30 am on a busy Monday morning it may be difficult for a stressed receptionist to make an incoming caller feel 'welcome' – difficult, but not impossible. It may be helpful to have some kind of personal motto to say to yourself at difficult times, such as 'Do as you would be done by' or 'Speak as you would want to be spoken to'. Self-control, conscious use of a warm tone of voice, and the personal motto are useful aids to ensuring that the telephone is answered to a consistently high standard.

Telephone enquiries

Secretaries and receptionists receive numerous telephone enquiries during the course of their day-to-day work. They may be typing lengthy reports, running a busy surgery or clinic or retrieving data from the computer, but the telephone enquiries and requests continue! Maintaining the balance between conflicting demands is part of the job, and the telephone caller should never have the impression that you are too flustered or annoyed at being interrupted and too busy to deal with their request.

- Answer the telephone as promptly as possible.

- Announce the name of the practice or clinic, and give your name (you will no doubt have your protocol for this).

- Establish the caller's identity and try to help.

- If the caller is using a pay-phone, take the number and ring them back promptly if necessary.

- Politely ask the caller to hold if you need to deal with a visitor.

Golden rules when using the telephone

- Be polite.

- Do not eat while you are speaking on the telephone.

- Do not hold two conversations at the same time.

- Return to the caller every 30 seconds if you are keeping them on hold.

- If you are unable to help the caller yourself, track down someone who can – if necessary call them back.

People skills – face to face

In contrast to telephone communication, where the only indicators are words and tone of voice, in a face-to-face encounter there is the additional dimension of 'non-verbal communication'. This consists of the signals that are given out and picked up, sometimes subconsciously, but which cause a reaction every bit as strong as that to the words and tone of voice. For example, a patient who is failing to get what they want is not only likely to raise their voice, but may well lean forward over the reception counter. In response, the receptionist could either spontaneously lean forward with a matching aggressive reaction, step back from the desk in a defensive manner, or calmly remain in the same position. Not only does the body move and thereby speak more clearly than our words, but the hands and face highlight the expression of feeling. For example, hands may become clenched into fists and smiles disappear. With this knowledge in mind, the skill is to maintain self-control and gain control of the situation. There are no set patterns for dealing with difficult situations, but attending courses, practice in role play, watching video clips, discussing situations after they have occurred, watching colleagues and learning from their successes/ weaknesses can all contribute to gaining experience and improving existing skills.

The medical receptionist or secretary also needs constantly to bear in mind the fact that patients are likely to feel unwell, be anxious about what is going to be done to them and what the doctor may say, and concerned about the effect of their illness on their family. These feelings make patients stressed and therefore more sensitive to offhand treatment. From the moment they are dealt with they need to feel that they are the one and only concern of the receptionist.

Box 3.4

Recall good and bad experiences of how you have been made to feel in shops, offices, hospital and the doctor's surgery.

What made you feel bad?

What made you feel good?

What can you incorporate into your way of working to make patients feel as good as they can in the circumstances?

Meetings

Staff meetings, departmental or primary healthcare team meetings and patient participation groups are the type of meeting where receptionists and secretaries may be required to express a view. With modern management techniques, meetings have become an important tool for communication. They provide the opportunity to find out what is going on, to be updated with the latest information and to contribute to forward planning. Even in a well-chaired, relatively informal meeting, staff who have every confidence in dealing with difficult patients at the desk may find it almost impossible to speak out in a meeting with doctors and/or managers present. Skill in speaking out can be cultivated by practice and helped by planning.

Box 3.5

If you are going to be called upon to speak, prepare for the occasion.

DO

Read the agenda circulated a few days before the meeting.

Think about what you want to say.

Write down a few key words.

Define one statement that encapsulates your view succinctly.

Make an outline of what you want to say.

You should succeed in confidently making your point and gain respect not only for your view, but for your ability to communicate.

DON'T

Go into the meeting intending to say whatever comes into your head at the time.

You may lose the opportunity to say what you really want to say, waste other people's time, and they may lose respect for you.

Performance review

Receptionists and secretaries will no doubt be aware of other forms of 'communication' within their organisations, such as performance review or 'appraisal' interviews, where they will be given the opportunity to communicate how they perceive their personal strengths and limitations, and perhaps identify areas where further training is needed.

Counselling

Counselling may be defined as: 'assisting individuals towards independence or self-actualisation'. It is a form of communication that is designed to enable employees to make their own decisions or choices. It involves:

- listening
- guiding
- communicating
- information giving.

Counselling is non-judgemental, does not make assumptions, and can be used either to prevent a problem, or to help to work through an existing problem.

The practice leaflet

Practice information leaflets communicate to patients the services available at the practice and how they may make better use of the primary healthcare service. New patients will find the practice leaflet a valuable source of information, not only about the services offered, but also about the members of the primary healthcare team, the times of the surgery and clinic sessions, and how to contact the doctor in an emergency.

Your practice leaflets should be attractively designed to make both patients and potential patients aware of the services and quality of care provided. They should be prominently positioned on the reception counter and readily accessible to all callers.

Hospital information leaflets

NHS trusts and private hospitals and clinics will provide information about the services which they offer. As well as basic information about hospital clinics, open-access facilities and times of visiting, etc., they will give details of transport to the hospital and car-parking facilities.

Networking

Every organisation is changing to a greater or lesser degree on a regular basis. Staff come and go, the organisational structure changes, and responsibilities are shifted from one department to another. Therefore it is important that personal contacts are made and maintained so that if a receptionist/secretary does not know how to do something, or does not have a vital piece of information, then there is always someone to turn to who will either know the answer themselves or 'know a man who does'. It is also important to keep up to date with the latest information by reading magazines as a vital supplement to networking.

Barriers to communication

Physical barriers

Physical barriers to communication may include the following:

- too much noise
- insufficient privacy
- frequent interruptions
- physical handicap (e.g. deafness, blindness or stammer)
- the reception counter being either too high or too low
- telephone constantly ringing.

Receptionists'/secretaries' language

The language used when speaking to patients is a vital part of good communication. You must be aware of:

- using words (and 'jargon') that the patient cannot understand
- talking too quickly or too quietly
- talking with a strong accent
- confusing patients by giving them too much information.

Patients' language

Patients from ethnic minorities may have difficulty in understanding and speaking the English language. You may have a colleague who can speak their language, or an interpreter may be necessary.

Psychological barriers

You must be aware of the psychological elements which may form barriers to good communication. Patients may find it difficult to communicate for the following reasons:

- feelings of inadequacy

- lack of confidence

- being emotionally upset by pain and/or anxiety about their medical condition

- being unable to concentrate because of illness.

Attitudes of secretaries and receptionists

Remember the importance of positive non-verbal signs. A negative attitude will be a barrier to communication, for example:

- being impatient and rude

- not giving one's undivided attention

- appearing critical or demonstrating a superior attitude

- avoiding eye contact

- appearing to be too busy

- feeling irritated and under stress.

Attitudes of patients

An understanding of the reasons for patients' attitudes may help you to deal with them in a sympathetic manner and to overcome the barrier that their attitude may present. For example, they may be:

- too ill to concentrate

- resentful at having to present themselves at the reception desk

- terrified that they may have a serious illness

- afraid of appearing stupid to the efficient secretary or receptionist

- struggling with a personal problem

- inhibited by finding that they know the receptionist or secretary socially.

Overcoming the barriers

An awareness of the barriers, combined with good common sense, is a good start to overcoming any problems.

*   Try to answer all questions in a positive way.

*   A pleasant manner, a smile and understanding often do the trick – it is hard to be difficult when empathy is extended to one.

*   Always be polite.

*   Be alert to any problems which might occur.

*   Always try to be helpful, smiling, calm and able to cope.

*   If patients are kept waiting for longer than is necessary, apologise and give an explanation.

*   When making appointments, ensure that the patient has the date and time written down to avoid any future misunderstanding.

*   Try to give each patient your attention when dealing with them. Make eye contact and listen carefully to what they are saying.

*   Never sound tired or bored, or look as if you are not listening.

Confidentiality

Remember that the rules of confidentiality that apply to working in any healthcare environment are just as important when communicating with patients.

All information is privileged information, and *must not* be divulged without the doctor's prior consent.

4

Law, ethics and medicine

Introduction

The relationships between professional healthcare workers and between them and their patients are governed by the professional ethics and etiquette of medicine which have developed over the centuries, together with developments in medicine itself. Secretaries and receptionists working closely with doctors and other healthcare workers, as well as being in constant communication with patients, should be aware of the important role of ethics and etiquette.

Ethics relate to moral principles and standards of what is morally right and wrong, and are the guiding rules of professional behaviour. They are directed towards the benefit of the patients. *Etiquette* is concerned with the courtesy and politeness of normal behaviour.

History of ethics and etiquette

History shows that even from the earliest times, various legal systems have incorporated some degree of regulation of doctors. The earliest records were the Code of Laws of Hammurabi (1790 BC), when fees were regulated. Success was rewarded in accordance with the status of the patient, but failure was punished, frequently by mutilation.

The earliest record and declaration of ethics was made in the Hippocratic Oath (400 BC), which reflects the culture of the Hippocratic physicians. The standards expressed in the Hippocratic Oath, although no longer affirmed by today's physicians, are still accepted as the ideal of professional behaviour (*see* Appendix 2).

The Hippocratic Oath demonstrates the early concern of the profession to regulate itself by laying down basic standards of professional conduct, not only between doctor and patient, but also between teacher and pupil. For centuries thereafter, the principles of Christian humanism dominated the practice of medicine. Traditions of etiquette in public and private life gradually developed and, combined with the criteria of professional conduct, established the physician's position in society.

In 1798, the proposals of Sir Thomas Percival in Manchester ultimately became the *Professional Conduct of Physicians and Surgeons*, published in 1803. This laid down the foundations for modern ethical standards in the UK.

The Provincial Medical and Surgical Association that was formed in 1832, and which became the British Medical Association (BMA) in 1856, appointed a committee on medical ethics in 1849. This formed the basis of the General Ethical Committee of the BMA, which has always played a leading role not only in establishing ethical standards for the professional in the UK, but also in setting standards adopted as norms of conduct for doctors in many parts of the world.

The BMA was largely responsible for the establishment of the General Medical Council (GMC) under the Medical Act of 1858. The GMC has a regulatory role, and from time to time issues guidance to members of the medical profession to enable them to avoid action which might lead to charges of professional misconduct. (The roles of both the BMA and the GMC will be covered in more detail later in this chapter.)

Medical ethics and etiquette

Every medical receptionist and secretary must be aware of the important areas of ethical behaviour and etiquette. It has already been stated that ethics are directed towards the benefit of the patients, and many are bound into a code of conduct published by the GMC for doctors, and by other regulatory bodies for other health professionals, for example:

- the General Dental Council (GDC)

- the United Kingdom Central Council for Nursing, Midwifery and Health Visiting (UKCC).

The GDC maintains a register of dentists, and promotes high standards of dental education as well as standards of professional conduct among dentists. It also has disciplinary powers with regard to the professional conduct of dentists.

The UKCC is the regulatory body which sets standards for the education and conduct of the nursing, widwifery and health-visiting professions. It also maintains the professional registers.

All regulatory bodies have the responsibility of maintaining the register of those allowed to practise as doctors, dentists, nurses, etc. The ultimate sanction on those judged to have behaved unethically is the removal of their names from the register, and thus the removal of their ability to practise.

There are no formal sanctions for those in breach of etiquette, but the rules have been established by custom. They aid communication between professionals and avoid damaging reputations, so they may be said to benefit patients indirectly.

A modern restatement of the Hippocratic Oath was formulated by the World Medical Association in 1947 to reflect the changing attitudes of society and major advances in medical science. It is known as the Declaration of Geneva:

> I solemnly pledge myself to consecrate my life to the service of humanity;
> I will give to my teachers the respect and gratitude which is their due;
> I will practise my profession with dignity;
> The health of my patient will be my first consideration;
> I will respect the secrets which are confided in me, even after the patient has died;
> I will maintain by all the means of my power, the honour and the noble traditions of the medical profession;
> My colleagues will be my brothers;
> I will not permit considerations of religion, nationality, race, party politics or social standing to intervene between me and my patients;
> I will maintain the utmost respect for human life from the time of conception; even under threat I will not use my medical knowledge contrary to the laws of humanity;
> I make these promises solemnly, freely and upon my honour.

There are four important areas of ethical behaviour and etiquette of which all secretaries and receptionists in medical practice should be aware, and the principles of which they should apply to their day-to-day work. These areas are:

- confidentiality

- trust

- confidence

- integrity.

Confidentiality

Confidentiality places a constraint upon all those who work in the field of healthcare. The terms and conditions of employment of medical secretaries and receptionists, wherever employed, will almost certainly contain a clause to the effect that any breach of confidentiality will result in disciplinary action, or even dismissal. They will no doubt be asked to sign statements signifying that this is fully understood.

The Declaration of Geneva maintains that a doctor must preserve secrecy in all that he or she knows – even after the death of his or her patient. However, there are certain exceptions to this:

- when the patient gives consent

- when it is undesirable on medical grounds to seek a patient's consent, but it is in the patient's best interests that confidentiality should be broken

- the doctor's overriding duty to society

- for the purposes of medical research, when approved by a local clinical research ethical committee or, in the case of the National Cancer Registry, by the Chairman of the BMA's Central Ethical Committee.

Doctors must be able to justify their decisions to disclose information. A doctor must ensure, as far as possible, that all medical information is kept in a secure place.

Confidentiality and medical records

Secretaries and receptionists are in the privileged position of having access to medical records which contain confidential information about patients, and they should always remember that patients trust doctors not to divulge any personal information which is contained in the records. Likewise, confidential information should never be discussed or divulged by secretaries or receptionists.

Discretion is necessary when dealing with enquiries from solicitors, relatives or representatives of the patient, and insurance companies. Staff should always be circumspect when they are dealing with patients. When speaking with colleagues, great care should be taken. Some hospitals insist that patients are referred to by their hospital number and not by their name.

Secretaries and receptionists working in a hospital will usually find that their medical records manager will require them to sign a form stating that they understand the legal and ethical aspects of confidentiality, and that any behaviour contravening this may result in termination of employment.

Any information that is contained in medical records may only be disclosed in certain circumstances.

Trust

As part of their work in dealing with patients and their families, doctors are entrusted with information that would not be divulged to others. Good medical practice is based on the maintenance of trust between doctors, patients and their families, with the knowledge that professional relationships will be strictly observed. Not only doctors, but also medical secretaries and receptionists must at all times exercise care and discretion to maintain this special relationship.

Confidence

Confidence, like trust, is also vitally important in the doctor–patient relationship. Staff should appreciate that if patients have been helped by a doctor on a previous occasion, they are confident that they will be helped in any further episodes. Although this may make the doctor's task easier, it also places added responsibility on him or her, as doctors know they cannot always succeed.

The trust and confidence which patients should ideally have in their physicians and surgeons provides them with the will to overcome illness and make a good recovery. It is important to appreciate that when people are ill they want to see doctors and their staff who treat them with kindness and consideration, and who respect their views and feelings.

Integrity

Doctors will act professionally and objectively in the best interests of their patients in their judgements and patient care. Receptionists and staff should also behave in a professional manner and remain circumspect at all times. Considerable pressure is placed on doctors and healthcare staff (e.g. by relatives, advertising, the media, etc.). It is perhaps worth considering the duties of a doctor and the rights of patients in the context of ethics and etiquette in medicine.

Doctors' duties

At the end of 1996, the GMC published *Duties of a Doctor*, which describes good medical practice and gives guidance on the duties of doctors registered with the GMC. Patients must be able to trust doctors with their lives and well-being. To justify that trust, they as a profession have a duty to maintain a good standard of practice and care and to show respect for human life. In particular, doctors must:

- make the care of their patients their first concern
- treat every patient politely and considerately
- respect patients' dignity and privacy
- listen to patients and respect their views
- give patients information in a form that they can understand
- respect the rights of patients to be fully involved in decisions about their care
- keep their professional knowledge and skills up to date
- recognise the limits of their professional competence
- be honest and trustworthy
- respect and protect confidential information
- make sure that their personal beliefs do not prejudice their patients' care
- act quickly to protect patients from risk if they have good reason to believe that they or a colleague may not be fit to practise
- avoid abusing their position as doctors
- work with colleagues in the ways that best serve patients' interests.

In all of these matters, doctors must never discriminate against their patients or colleagues, and must always be prepared to justify their actions to them.

Overall management

It is good medical practice for one doctor to be responsible for the overall management of a particular patient's illness.

Referral from a GP to a consultant has evolved in the patient's interest. A consultant or specialist should not accept a patient without referral from a GP, although there are exceptions (e.g. sexually transmitted diseases, family planning and casualty).

Consent to treatment

The patient's trust that their consent to treatment will not be abused is an essential part of their relationship with their doctor. For a doctor even to touch a patient without their consent constitutes an assault. Doctors offer advice, but it is the patient who decides whether or not to accept that advice. It is the doctor's duty of care to give advice about the significant facts and inherent risks to a patient, so that the patient understands the nature of the proposed treatment and is able to give their consent.

Patients' rights

Patients have certain rights with regard to their use of healthcare services. These rights generally fall into two categories:

1   the right to treatment
2   the right to confidentiality.

The right to treatment

All patients:

- have the right to be on a GP's list of patients
- have the right to see a GP (not necessarily their own doctor) at the GP's surgery at any time during surgery hours
- should have access to a telephone number at which a GP can be reached 24 hours a day, 365 days a year
- should be visited at home if it is considered necessary by the GP
- must receive any treatment which is immediately necessary when they are temporarily away from home

- have the right to change GPs without giving a reason, by applying to another GP

- have no absolute right to a second opinion, but the doctor should take reasonable care to seek one if they are unsure of the diagnosis or treatment

- need to give consent before being examined or treated

- are not legally bound to accept treatment. However, doctors can give essential treatment if the patient is temporarily incapable of under-standing or consenting to treatment (e.g. due to alcohol or drugs). If the patient is permanently incapable due to mental illness, it is poss-ible for a legal guardian to give consent

- have the right to refuse to be examined with a medical student present

- have the right to a full and truthful reply to any specific question unless the information may result in anxiety which could injure the patient's health

- have the right to see and amend medical records made on or after 1 November 1991, unless they will cause harm to the patient (*see* Access to Health Records Act 1990). Hospitals, private clinics, GP practices, etc. who hold patient information on computer have to conform to the Data Protection Act, which protects patients' rights (*see* Data Protection Act 1984)

- have the right to complain about their doctor if they have not followed their terms of service, or if a doctor behaves in an unethical manner.

The right to confidentiality

Doctors must not pass on information without the patient's consent except to those involved in their treatment and care or, when it is in the best interests of the patient, to close relatives. The law requires doctors to give information about patients to health and other authorities in the following circumstances:

- when ordered by a court

- if the patient has certain infectious diseases or food poisoning

- if they suspect that the patient is addicted to a 'hard' drug

- if they arrange an abortion for a patient

- if required by the police to help to identify a driver suspected of motoring offences.

Chaperoning

All too frequently we hear about doctors being accused of indecently assaulting their patients, and doctors today are at risk from such accusations. The presence of a third person as a chaperone, usually a nurse, is a valuable insurance for the practitioner. However, there may be occasions when the doctor's secretary or receptionist will be asked to be present at the consultation, particularly in private practice when a nurse is not always available.

On some occasions, a chaperone is requested, particularly by an elderly woman or a woman from an ethnic minority (where removing a veil in the presence of a male person who is not a member of the family is an uncommon occurrence). Any requests, particularly of a cultural origin, should always be treated with great respect.

The presence of a chaperone for unaccompanied children or patients with a mental disorder is often requested, not only for the protection of the doctor, but also in very exceptional circumstances for that of the patient.

It is considered that chaperones are advisable, but it may be that one is not always available when required. Doctors normally exercise their discretion when requesting a chaperone, and are naturally very cautious as patients of both sexes have made complaints of indecent assault, and these are not necessarily limited to allegations against a doctor of the opposite sex.

If you are not comfortable in the role of chaperone, you should let your colleagues know, so that someone else will be available should the need arise.

If the patient is emotionally upset or mentally disturbed when consulting a doctor, the presence of a chaperone not only protects the doctor, but may also relieve the patient of some embarrassment and anxiety.

Consent to treatment

Patients' rights are an area of continuing concern for doctors and patients alike, particularly with regard to the controversial issue of 'informed consent'. As a medical receptionist or secretary, you should remember that doctors always require signed agreement from patients:

- before carrying out surgery and/or procedures

- prior to involving patients in clinical trials

- before publishing medical photographs for medical data, either in print or in data form.

Consent becomes 'informed consent' when patients are made fully aware of the risks, consequences or alternatives of any such treatment or procedure, and the risks involved in signing any form of consent. Doctors and other health professionals should tell patients about the complications of the procedure and the likelihood of its success. It should be ensured that the patient fully understands the explanation and has the opportunity to ask any questions, close relatives being involved if necessary.

Consent is only valid if the patient understands what their treatment involves and agrees to it.

Patients may choose whether or not to take part in medical student teaching or medical research, and may refuse to allow their consent to this.

The consent of the woman involved in termination of pregnancy and the consent of the physician is no longer necessary.

Similarly, a partner's consent to sterilisation is not legally required, but in accordance with Department of Health recommendations, doctors will usually want to consult the partner.

Children and young people

Children aged 16 years and over can normally consent to their own treatment. Young children under the age of 16 years may be able to consent if they are sufficiently mature to fully understand what is being proposed. However, in some instances (e.g. termination of pregnancy) a doctor will also require parental consent.

Mental health and consent

Mental health patients who are not detained under a section of the Mental Health Act (1983) have the same rights to consent as if they were receiving treatment for any physical illness. However, for patients detained under section, the situation is different in that their consent should be sought, but some treatment can be given without the patient's consent.

The regulatory bodies and their role

The General Medical Council

The General Medical Council (GMC) was established under the Medical Act of 1858 with the purpose of distinguishing between unqualified practitioners or 'quacks' and qualified medical practitioners. The Medical Register was thus established, which contains records of medical practitioners and their qualifications.

The GMC licenses doctors to practise in the UK under the provisions of the Medical Act of 1983. Its purpose is to ensure that the public is served by doctors who have the qualities it expects, and to protect them from doctors whose conduct, professional performance or health places patients at risk (General Medical Council: *Protecting Patients, Guiding Doctors*).

One of the most important functions of the GMC is to protect patients and to guide doctors.

Functions of the GMC

- The GMC keeps a register of all medical practitioners who have obtained qualifying degrees, giving them licence to practise. The GMC publishes this register, providing the public with the names of doctors who have acquired the necessary medical qualifications and experience to equip them to practise in the UK.

- It keeps a separate register of those practitioners who have obtained higher degrees.

- It sets out standards of medical education.

- It is responsible for the publication of the *British Pharmacopoeia* (*BP*).

- It has an important regulatory role in that it issues guidelines to all members of the medical profession to enable them to avoid actions which might lead to charges of professional misconduct.

- It has a duty to administer discipline. It is to the GMC that the public and medical profession may make complaints about a doctor's behaviour.

- It has the power, if such a charge is proved, to temporarily suspend a doctor from practising or, if necessary, to remove their name from ('strike them off') the register.

The GMC has influenced radical reform to medical regulation since 1858, a development which reflects modern medicine, its culture and the need for a new professionalism, but is also influenced by public expectations. When people are ill they want to see doctors who are skilful and who will treat them with kindness and consideration and respect their views.

> *Modernisation is needed, so that the GMC feels able to move quickly to suspend, remove or otherwise discipline doctors who are falling below the standards patients can expect, and to bring itself into the twenty-first century in terms of corporate governance and sensible decision making.*
>
> (Julia Neuberger, GMC lay member)

January 2000 saw the publication of new competence standards for general practitioners. Those doctors who do not reach the required standards may have to undergo retraining or even be prevented from treating the public. Dr Harold Shipman (who was found guilty of murdering many of his patients in February 2000 and was erased from the Register) and other cases have highlighted areas for reform, and the GMC has asked for greater powers to suspend doctors under investigation.

Doctors must be able to demonstrate to the GMC on a regular basis that they are up to date in their knowledge and skills, and are fit to practise in their chosen field of medicine. Together with clinical governance, it will be appreciated that much is being done to protect the public from unskilled practitioners.

Health procedures

In addition to conduct procedures, the GMC's health procedures look into the cases of doctors who are suffering from illnesses which affect their ability to practise medicine safely. These illnesses are almost invariably alcohol or drug related or a mental condition. The health procedures not only protect the public but also offer doctors expert medical supervision and support.

Performance procedures

In September 1997, the GMC's powers were extended to cover a third set of procedures to take action against incompetent doctors who represent a danger to their patients. Doctors referred to these procedures will have their professional performance assessed by teams of medical and lay assessors – the Committee on Professional Performance. If it is deemed appropriate, doctors will be asked to accept further training or counselling to remedy their deficiencies before an act of serious professional misconduct occurs.

Doctors whose performance is considered to be a serious risk to the public, or who are unwilling or unable to be retrained, will face a private hearing with the possibility of their registration being restricted or suspended.

The British Medical Association

The British Medical Association (BMA) was founded in 1832 by Charles Hastings, and it is the largest medical association in the UK. It is concerned with most aspects of medicine and is one of the principal bodies representing UK doctors.

The BMA played an important part in the establishment of the General Medical Council. The Ethics Department of the BMA plays a leading role in establishing ethical standards in the medical profession. It examines and advises on the increasing number of ethical matters in medical practice, and on the relationship between doctor and patient. The BMA issues guidelines on various ethical issues including the following:

* euthanasia

* genetic counselling

* surrogacy.

The BMA publishes one of the world's leading medical journals, the *British Medical Journal*, which covers many topics of concern and interest to the medical profession, including original papers on clinical, scientific, political and social subjects.

Medical science is advancing rapidly and, with new discoveries being communicated to the public, the BMA issues ethical guidelines that reflect and safeguard the well-being and interests of patients, and at the same time express the views of the profession on medical ethics.

Summary of medical ethics and etiquette

In looking at the ethics and etiquette of medical practice, the medical receptionist or secretary will understand that patients expect doctors not only to use their expertise and skill, but also to observe absolute confidentiality with regard to any information that is imparted as a result of the consultation, examination and treatment. On this understanding of professional confidence and secrecy, all of those working in the field of healthcare will be aware of the special relationship which exists between doctor and patient.

Having considered the various ethical issues that confront the medical profession, and the role of the regulatory bodies, we are now able to appreciate the problems facing doctors and their ability to resolve the numerous ethical and moral dilemmas that may arise. These include the following:

- abortion
- euthanasia
- screening
- genetic counselling
- artificial insemination
- severely malformed infants
- *in-vitro* fertilisation
- consent to operations on reproductive organs
- HIV/AIDS
- euthanasia
- surrogacy
- transplantation
- the use of human tissue
- other issues arising from advances in biomedical and biological research.

Practical considerations for secretaries and receptionists

- Remember that your work is strictly confidential – anything that is divulged by a patient to the doctor, the medical records or correspondence, must not be disclosed to anyone else.
- Details of your work or personal affairs of doctors and other healthcare professionals must *not* be discussed.
- The behaviour of or treatment by a medical practitioner or any professional healthcare worker must *not* be openly criticised within hearing distance of the patient.
- Always be circumspect when talking about a doctor or other healthcare professional to another person. Do not unduly praise or criticise their accomplishments.
- It is your responsibility to facilitate the doctor's treatment and care of his or her patients.

Legal aspects

Medical secretaries and receptionists, although they do not need a detailed knowledge of law, should have an understanding of those legal aspects that affect their day-to-day work.

Patient access to information

Over the past decade, patients and carers have had an increasing expectation of access to information about their own healthcare, and this trend has been encouraged by NHS policy. There are very good reasons for giving patients access. First, it is ethical to do so, as truth-telling is not only a moral absolute but also produces a relationship based on mutual trust. Secondly, there is abundant evidence that people want more information about their own healthcare and treatment, and clinical trials have demonstrated that improved functional and health status is linked to good doctor–patient information sharing. Thirdly, legislation requires that patients should have access to information, and rights to information in the UK have since 1991 been set out in the Patient's Charter, which summarises the rights and standards based on both legislation and common law. The right of access to health records was established by two acts of Parliament:

- the Data Protection Act 1984
- the Access to Health Records Act 1990.

More recently, new agendas have emphasised the need for improved patient access to information, including the following:

- Purchasing Intelligence and Local Voice
- NHS Code of Openness
- Patient Partnership Strategy
- Promoting Clinical Effectiveness
- NHS Research and Development.

There is an increasing awareness that sharing information with patients, carers and the wider public can be a significant factor in encouraging informed and discerning use of health services. Sharing information also encourages professionals to develop skills in communicating with patients.

The NHS Code of Openness (published in 1995) encourages both purchasers and providers to enable public access to information about NHS organisations, including trusts and health authorities and, at the present time, community health councils. The public also have the right to attend certain meetings of NHS organisations, and have the opportunity to put forward their views, as part of a commitment to public consultation. This includes information about costs, quality and performance, proposed service changes and how to influence decisions and actions that affect their own treatment, and what information is available and how to obtain it. There has been a recent noticeable growth in information services for patients and the public. Under the Patient's Charter, a single national freephone number for health information was established and health service guidelines required local centres to provide information on the following:

- common illnesses and treatments
- self-help groups
- waiting-times
- healthcare services
- keeping healthy
- patients' rights and how to complain
- Patient's Charter standards.

Medical records

Hospitals, general practices and any healthcare organisations that record information on computer about identifiable living individuals must ensure that they comply with the provisions of the Data Protection Act.

The Data Protection Act 1984

The Data Protection Act is designed and based on principles to ensure that information relating to an individual is obtained fairly, kept up to date and stored securely. Individuals whose data are stored have rights of access enabling them to check the accuracy of the information. The data protection registrar and the courts are empowered to require correction of inaccurate material if it is not undertaken voluntarily by the data user.

The medical context of the individual's right of access to information held about him or her has been modified by the Data Protection (Subject Access Modification) (Health) Order 1987. This allows information to be withheld from an individual if it is likely to cause serious harm to his or her mental or physical health, or if it discloses the identity of a person other than the healthcare professional. A doctor who withholds information must be prepared to justify his or her actions in a court if challenged at a later date. This Act applies to England, Wales, Scotland and Northern Ireland.

The Access to Medical Reports Act 1988

This Act establishes an individual's right of access to medical reports prepared for insurance or employment purposes by doctors who either are, or have been, responsible for that person's care. The Act applies only to England, Wales and Scotland, but similar provisions now apply to Northern Ireland under the Access to Personal Files and Medical Reports Order 1991.

At the same time that the patient's consent to the preparation of the report is obtained, the commissioning company is required to inform the individual of his or her rights under the Act, and to enquire whether access to the report is required. The information is then passed on to the doctor.

If the patient requires access, he or she is allowed 21 days to make appropriate arrangements to view the report. Patients who originally declined the opportunity of access may make an application to see the report until the time it is despatched to the company and, if so, must be allowed 21 days to make appropriate arrangements.

Once the report has been seen by the patient, he or she may agree to the despatch unaltered, request correction of factual accuracy or, if the doctor declines to make the requested correction, append a statement of their own, or they may refuse to allow the report to be released.

The Human Rights Act (1988)

The Human Rights Act incorporates the European Convention on Human Rights (ECHR) into English law. It brings with it new responsibilities for all who work in public authorities. Our courts now have to take into account the case law of the European court.

The main aim of the Act is to allow the rights given under the European Convention on Human Rights (ECHR) of 1950, and the Act will contribute towards a society where the rights and responsibilities of individuals are carefully considered and where awareness of the rights of the ECHR permeate government and legal systems.

A 'public authority' includes the following:

* central government
* local government
* the courts
* police.

It also includes many other bodies who carry out functions which the Government would otherwise have to undertake, including health authorities and trusts, local authorities, government agencies, Courts and tribunals. Any person or organisation that carries out some functions of a public nature is also included, although under the Act they are only considered to be a public authority in relation to their public functions.

All public authorities have a positive obligation to ensure that respect for human rights is at the core of their day-to-day work, which means that they should act in a way that positively reinforces the principles of the Act. This is further emphasised by the fact that it is unlawful for a public authority to act (or fail to act) in a way which is incompatible with an ECHR right. This includes the following aspects of the activities of a public authority:

- drafting rules and regulations
- internal staff and personnel issues
- administrative procedures
- decision making
- policy implementation
- interaction with members of the public.

At the very core of every organisation there should be respect for EHCR rights, and if existing procedures are not compatible, new policies and procedures will have to be implemented.

In their day-to-day work, public authority officials should always act in accordance with the ECHR rights in demonstrating a positive attitude to human rights.

The Access to Health Records Act 1990

This Act applies to England, Wales and Scotland and has established a right of access for patients to whom the records relate and, in certain circumstances, to other individuals. The Act also makes provision for correction of inaccurate records.

Under the Act, a health record is any record containing information relating to the physical or mental health of an individual who can be identified from that information which has been made by 'or on behalf of' a healthcare professional.

Applications for access must be made in writing to the record holder and, provided that no addition to the record has been made within the previous 40 days, a fee may be charged. Provided that there is no reason to withhold access, the record holder must allow the applicant to see the records within 40 days, unless the most recent note has been made within 40 days, in which case the time limit is 21 days. If a copied set of the medical record is required, a copying and postal charge may be made. Applications may be made by the patient or by someone appointed on the patient's behalf. This may be:

- in the case of a child, the parent or guardian

- in the case of an incapable patient, a person appointed by the court to manage the patient's affairs

- after a patient's death, the patient's personal representatives or anyone who might have a claim arising out of the patient's death.

The law and mental health

Mental Health Act

Secretaries and receptionists working in the field of healthcare will need an understanding of the implications of the law relating to mental illness.

The law changed with the Mental Health Act of 1983. The provisions of this Act are of particular importance to those patients who are compulsorily detained under the Act. This involves approximately 10% of all patients who are admitted to psychiatric hospitals or departments.

The Mental Health Act of 1983 established the Mental Health Act Commission, which has a responsibility to protect the rights of detained patients and to keep under review the exercise of compulsory power and duties conferred by the Act. The Act also provides the legal instrument which enables society to act in the interests of, and on behalf of, patients and those convicted of certain criminal offences who are diagnosed as having certain abnormal mental conditions, and makes provision for the protection of the public, and for the protection of the property of patients who are compulsorily detained.

The primary concerns of the 1983 Mental Health Act are:

- protection of the mentally ill patient

- protection of his or her property

- protection of the public.

The Act defines certain relevant legal mental conditions as follows.

- *Mental disorder* – which means illness, arrested or incomplete development of mind, psychopathic disorder or any other disorder or disability of mind.

- *Severe mental impairment* – which means a state of arrested or incomplete development of intelligence and social functioning, and is associated with abnormally aggressive or seriously irresponsible conduct on the part of the person concerned.

- *Mental impairment* – which means a state of arrested or incomplete development of mind (not amounting to severe mental impairment) which includes significant impairment of intelligence and social functioning, and is associated with abnormally aggressive or seriously irresponsible conduct on the part of the person concerned.

- *Psychopathic disorder* – which means a persistent disorder or disability of mind (whether or not it includes significant impairment of intelligence) which results in abnormally aggressive or seriously irresponsible conduct on the part of the person concerned.

A person may not be regarded as suffering from mental disorder by reason only of promiscuity or other immoral conduct, sexual deviancy or dependence on alcohol or drugs.

The legislation emphasises the following:

1 as much treatment as possible on a voluntary basis, both in hospital and in the home or other institution
2 a shift from institutional care to care within the home as far as is possible
3 proper provision for those to be detained on a compulsory basis in the interests of the patient and society.

Medical secretaries and receptionists will from time to time be involved in arrangements for patient admission, either formally or informally, to undergo psychiatric treatment. Such admissions come within sections of the Mental Health Act. A brief outline of admission under some of the sections of the Mental Health Act is given below.

Methods by which a person may enter a hospital for psychiatric treatment

Informal admission (Section 131)

Any person having attained the age of 16 years may request admission, or a person under the age of 16 years where the parent or guardian gives consent, or any person to whom it is suggested that admission is advisable and that person does not refuse, can be admitted without any legal formalities. This patient can discharge him or herself unless the doctor in charge decides that, if discharged, he or she would be endangering his or her health or safety or that of others.

Compulsory admission and detention

The following methods of admission can be used when a person suffering from mental disorder as defined by the Act is in need of psychiatric care but is not prepared to enter hospital or remain in hospital for observation or treatment.

- *Section 2 (up to 28 days)*: Admission for assessment (or for assessment followed by medical treatment).
  An application for the admission of the patient must be made by either an approved social worker or the nearest relative, plus a medical recommendation from one 'psychiatrist' and a doctor (if practicable, one doctor should have previous acquaintance of the patient – for example, his or her GP). The person making the application should have seen the patient within the last 14 days.

- *Section 3 (up to six months)*: Detention for treatment.
  The application for detention under Section 3 is the same as that for Section 2, except that the approved social worker is not to act if the nearest relative objects. This section can be reviewed for a further six months, and yearly thereafter.

  Note: Patients may apply to the Mental Health Review Tribunal (MHRT) under Sections 2 and 3, subject to the stated criteria.

- *Section 4 (up to 72 hours)*: Admission for assessment.
  The application must be made by either an approved social worker or the nearest relative, plus a recommendation from a medical practitioner who must have seen the patient within the last 24 hours. The patient must arrive at the hospital within 24 hours of the medical examination. (This may be converted into Section 2 if a second medical recommendation is received within 72 hours.)

Consent to treatment

Certain sections (56–64) of the Mental Health Act are largely concerned with consent to treatment for long-term detained patients, but certain safeguards also apply to informal patients.

The Mental Health (Patients in the Community) Act 1995

The Mental Health (Patients in the Community) Act 1995, which came into force on 1 April 1996, introduced a new power of supervised discharge available in the case of unrestricted patients who, in the opinion of the responsible medical officer, are ready to leave hospital but, because of the risk they present to themselves or others, need special support to live safely in the community. The patient's care plan, which must be in place before an application for supervised discharge is made, may include formal requirements such as attendance for rehabilitation or treatment, or the requirement to live at a particular residence. A named supervisor and responsible medical officer will be identified. Non-compliance will lead to an immediate review and possible compulsory readmission.

Care Programme Approach

The Care Programme Approach (CPA) is one of the cornerstones of policy on mental health, providing a framework for the care of mentally ill people which ensures that services are targeted at people with severe mental health problems.

Building Bridges

This paper, which was published in November 1996, offers detailed advice and guidance on arrangements for effective, co-ordinated, inter-agency work for the care and protection of severely mentally ill people.

Reforming the Mental Health Act

The White Paper published in December 2000, *Reforming the Mental Health Act*, describes the Government's proposals for legal reforms to reflect changes in mental healthcare, in particular the increased use of treatment in the community.

The White Paper is divided into two parts. Part 1, entitled *The New Legal Framework*, explains how new mental health legislation will operate for patients generally. It outlines the following:

- a new broad definition of mental disorder*

- a new three-stage process for the use of compulsory powers

- a range of safeguards for patients' interests, including a new independent Mental Health Tribunal, a right to independent advocacy, a new Commission for Mental Health, and a statutory requirement to develop care plans

- new duties covering the disclosure of information about patients who are suffering from a mental disorder.

*A new broad definition of mental disorder covers any disability or disorder of mind or brain, whether permanent or temporary, that results in impairment or disturbance of mental functioning. The same criteria will be used to determine whether an individual falls within the scope of the legislation, whatever their diagnosis.

Part 2, entitled *High-Risk Patients*, sets out specific arrangements for individuals who are deemed to pose a significant risk of harm to others as a result of their disorder. It outlines the following:

- new criteria linking the use of compulsory powers to the availability of a treatment plan needed to treat the underlying mental disorder

- the establishment of new facilities for those who are dangerous and severely personality disordered (DSPD).

Employment law

There are a number of laws that influence the employment of staff. It is important that all employees, including medical secretaries and receptionists, understand their rights. The key pieces of legislation are noted at the end of this section in Table 4.1.

From the point when a verbal offer of a job has been made and the post accepted, the formal contract comes into being. At this stage nothing further is required to signify its existence and both parties are bound by it from that point on. However, to avoid any misunderstanding, employers will generally follow up a job offer and acceptance with a letter.

Written statement of main terms and conditions

Employers are required to provide employees who are working eight hours or more each week with a written statement of the main terms and conditions of their employment within two months of starting work. This was not the case prior to 1993, but if any such staff who were appointed before this date ask for a statement, they must be given one within two months of asking. All staff must be given notification of any changes to specified terms and conditions when they occur.

The written statement must contain the following information:

- employer's name
- employee's name
- the starting date of employment
- the date when continuous service began and whether or not employment with another employer (another hospital or medical practice) is counted

- job title
- rate of pay
- payment intervals (monthly, weekly)
- hours of work
- place of work
- holiday entitlement and holiday pay.

The following additional information must also be provided within the two-month period (as part of the principal statement or separately):

- sick leave and sick pay
- pension scheme
- notice periods on either side
- end date of a fixed-term contract, or likely end date of a temporary one
- particulars of collective agreements where these apply (e.g. as agreed by Whitley Council)
- grievance procedure and with whom a grievance can be raised
- disciplinary rules and procedures, and to whom appeals can be made (this applies only to employers of 20 or more staff).

Sometimes relevant information relating to sickness, pensions, grievances, disciplinary rules, procedures and appeals is kept in separate reference documents. In this case, the written statement will refer to these, and they should be readily accessible to employees in the course of their work.

Equality of opportunity

We discriminate between people both in the workplace and in day-to-day life. Some forms of discrimination are acceptable but others are not, and certain forms have been determined to be unlawful. Legislation relating to equality of opportunity requires employers to exercise some form of social responsibility in making decisions about current or potential employees. Employees, too, may unconsciously discriminate between people – we are not always aware of how our prejudices and preconceptions colour our judgement and the way in which we deal with others.

Equality can only be achieved through an acceptance by all members of the work team that it is important, in their own interests and in the interests of the service that they provide.

Equal opportunities legislation

Equality of opportunity regardless of sex, race, marital status, disablement, religion or age is vitally important, not only for employees to have a fair and equal chance of developing their potential abilities and realising their expectations, but also for employers to make full and effective use of their staff and to improve employee relations. This legislation forbids discrimination between men and women with regard to pay and other terms in their contracts. Examples are listed below.

1   *Equal Pay Act 1970 and Equal Pay (Amendments) Regulations 1983*:

* overtime
* bonus payments
* holiday and sick-pay entitlements.

2   *Rehabilitation of Offenders Act 1974*

This Act allows an individual who has had a conviction for an offence to put it behind them and be rehabilitated after a period of time. Their conviction becomes 'spent' and they may lawfully conceal it from a prospective employer as if it had never happened. However, certain exemptions exist.

3   *Sex Discrimination Act 1975*

This Act describes direct discrimination as occurring if, on the grounds of her sex, a woman is treated less favourably than a man would be treated.

4   *The Race Relations Act 1976 and the Race Relations (Amendment) Act 2000*

These Act forbids racial discrimination in employment and the provision of services. They state that no person should treat another less favourably on racial grounds, and they place a duty on public bodies to provide equality of opportunity.

5   *Disability Discrimination Act 1996*

This Act provides protection against discrimination for those who can show that they have a physical or mental impairment which has a substantial and long-term effect on their day-to-day activities. Employers are expected to make reasonable adjustments to the working environment where these will alleviate the disadvantages or risks faced by the handicapped employees or prospective employees. In cases of discrimination, tribunals or county courts can award compensation. There is no compensation limit.

General responsibilities under these Acts

Hospitals, medical practices, etc. have a legal obligation to ensure that they and their employees do not discriminate unlawfully.

All supervisory staff are responsible for eliminating any sexual harassment, victimisation or intimidation of which they are aware.

Individual employees are expected to co-operate with measures designed to ensure equal opportunities and avoid unlawful discrimination. They should be encouraged to report incidents of harassment, victimisation and pressure to discriminate where these occur.

Sexual harassment

Sexual harassment is judged as unlawful behaviour contrary to the Sex Discrimination Act 1974. Examples of sexual harassment include the following:

*   unwanted physical contact

*   requests for sexual favours

*   unwelcome sexual advances

*   continued suggestions for social activity outside of work after it has been made clear that such suggestions are not welcome

*   offensive flirtation, suggestive remarks, etc.

*   the display of pornographic or sexually suggestive pictures, etc.

*   leering, whistling or making sexually suggestive gestures

*   derogatory or degrading abuse or insults which are gender related

*   offensive comments about appearance or dress.

Working-time regulations

These have been in place since 1 October 2000, and they provide new basic rights and protection for many workers, ensuring that they do not have to work excessive hours. In addition, they give rights to four weeks of paid holiday entitlement.

Part-time work regulations

From 1 July 2000 new regulations came into force for the purpose of ensuring that individuals in part-time employment are treated no less favourably than those in full-time employment.

Support for parents, families and carers

Legislation to support women in maternity has existed for many years, but a number of recent developments within the Employment Relations Act 1999 have extended support to parents and carers.

- *Time off for dependents*: This was introduced on 15 December 1999. All employees will have the right to take a reasonable period of time off work in order to deal with an emergency involving a dependent.

- *Parental leave directive*: Again as from 15 December 1999, this provides a right to parents of up to 13 weeks' unpaid leave, for individuals who meet the conditions within the regulations.

- *Maternity leave regulations*: These were amended on 30 April 2000. Leave was increased to 18 weeks and the qualifying service for additional maternity leave will decrease from two years to one year.

Table 4.1 Schedule of current employment legislation

Access to Medical Records Act 1988

Control of Substances Hazardous to Health Regulations 1988 (COSHH)

Data Protection Acts 1984 and 1988

Disability Discrimination Act 1995

Disabled Persons (Employment) Acts 1944 and 1958

Employment Acts 1980, 1982, 1989

Employment Protection Act 1975

Employment Protection (Consolidation) Act 1978 (EPCA)

Employment Relations Act 1999

Employment Rights (Dispute Resolution) Act 1996

Employment Tribunals Act 1996

Equal Pay Act 1970

Equal Pay (Amendment) Regulations 1983

Health and Safety (Display Screen Equipment) Regulations 1992

Health and Safety at Work Act 1974

Human Rights Act 1999

Management of Health and Safety at Work Regulations 1992

Manual Handling Operations Regulations 1992

Maternity Allowance and Statutory Maternity Pay Regulations 1994

National Minimum Wage Act 1998

Parental Leave Directive 1999

Part-time Workers Directive 2000

Personal Protective Equipment at Work Regulations 1992

Protection of Children Act 1999

Provision and Use of Work Equipment Regulations 1992

Public Interest Disclosure Act 1998

Race Relations Act 1976

Race Relations (Amendment) Act 2000

Rehabilitation of Offenders Act 1974 and Exceptions Order 1979

Sex Discrimination Act 1975

Social Security Act 1986

Social Security Contributions Benefits Act 1992

Statutory Sick Pay Act 1994

Trade Union and Labour Relations (Consolidation) Act 1993 (TULR[C]A)

Trade Union Reform and Employment Rights Act 1993

Transfer of Undertakings (Protection of Employment) Regulations 1981 (TUPE)

Unfair Contracts Terms Act 1977

Wages Act 1986

Working Time Regulations 1998

Workplace (Health Safety and Welfare) Regulations 1992

Certification

All doctors, whether they are working in private practices or in an NHS organisation, are from time to time requested to issue certificates, including the following:

- National Insurance/DSS certificates
- death certificates
- cremation certificates
- private medical or insurance certificates
- certificates of stillbirth.

Certification is a statutory obligation that is imposed upon doctors, and the secretary or receptionist should do all that they can to ensure that the doctor is not placed in the position of being asked to certify improperly.

For example, the doctor must always see the patient when issuing and signing the form on which a patient claims sickness benefit – Form Med 3 and 5 (*see* Figures 4.1 and 4.2). This should not be issued more than one day after examination, as the doctor has to certify that he or she has examined the patient today/yesterday.

Death certificates

The death certificate is the oldest of all official medical forms and is only issued to registered practitioners. The certificate is obtained from the registrar for the subdistrict in which the doctor practises. The issue of death certificates is a statutory requirement and no fee is chargeable. The certificate is given by a doctor who was actually attending the patient in their last illness, and where there is sufficient knowledge of the cause of death to do so. Doctors are bound by law to provide the certificate in a sealed envelope. The death certificate should be taken to the Registrar of Births and Deaths in the subdistrict of occurrence within five days of death.

There is no legal duty to notify the coroner of any death, but of course this does not imply that the doctor need not do so when the circumstances require such action. Moral, ethical and traditional considerations necessitate that the doctor acts with responsibility and, by notifying the coroner, facilitates any enquiry into the death as the coroner deems advisable.

Role of the medical secretary or receptionist

Secretaries and receptionists must appreciate that when dealing with grieving relatives, sympathy, understanding and patience will be required. They should ensure that the death certificate is available when required, and clearly explain what the relatives/representatives should do with it (e.g. take it to the registrar's office within the statutory time, and, if necessary, give them directions).

Cremation certificates

Doctors may be requested to sign cremation certificates for patients they have attended during their last illness. Cremation certificates require

---

FOR SOCIAL SECURITY AND STATUTORY SICK PAY PURPOSES ONLY

NOTES TO PATIENT ABOUT USING THIS FORM

You can use this form either:

1.   For Statutory Sick Pay (SSP) purposes - fill in Part A overleaf. Also fill in Part B if the doctor has given you a date to resume work. Give or send the completed form to your employer.

2.   For Social Security purposes -
To continue a claim for state benefit fill in parts A and C of the form overleaf. Also fill in Part B if the doctor has given you a date to resume work. Sign and date the form and give or send it to your Local Social Security Office QUICKLY to avoid losing benefit.

NOTE: To start your claim for State benefit you must use form SC1 if you are self-employed, unemployed or non-employed OR form SSP1 if you are an employee. For further details get leaflet IB202 (from Social Security Local Offices).

Doctor's Statement

In confidence to
Mr/Mrs/Miss/Ms ....
I examined you today/yesterday and advised you that
(a) You need not   (b) you should refrain from work
     refrain from
     work   for*† ....

                            OR until ....

Diagnosis of your disorder
causing absence from work ....
Doctor's remarks

Doctor's   Date of
Signature   signing

	Form Med 3

NOTE TO DOCTOR*† *See inside front cover for notes on completion*

Figure 4.1   Form Med 3 (sample).

if you cannot fill this in yourself ask someone to do so and sign it for you.

A. TO BE COMPLETED IN ALL CASES - PLEASE USE BLOCK LETTERS

Surname Mr/Mrs/Miss/Ms

First names

Present address

Postcode

	Date	Month	Year
Date of birth			

National Insurance Number

Works or Clock Number or Department

B. If the doctor has given you a date to resume work

Date you intend to start (or seek) work for any employer or as a self-employed person

	Date	Month	Year
day			

For night shift workers only

Shift will begin at | Time | am/pm

and end next day at | Time | am/pm

C. FOR STATE BENEFIT CLAIMANTS ONLY

Full name and address of employer (if employed)

DECLARATION

I understand that if I give incorrect or incomplete information action may be taken against me.

I declare that because of incapacity I have not worked since the date of my last claim.

I also declare that my circumstances and those of my dependants are and have been as last stated. (If there has been a change cross out this declaration and attach a signed and dated statement of new facts.)

I declare that the information I have given on this form is correct and complete.

I agree that the Department of Social Security or a doctor acting on their behalf may get in touch with my doctor so that they may give the Department of Social Security any information which is needed to deal with this claim and any request to look at the claim again.

Signature .... Date...

If you have signed this form for someone else please tick here

Printed for BA OSD/PCMG by Datasupplies 009000P 02/00

Figure 4.1   Continued.

FOR SOCIAL SECURITY AND STATUTORY   **Special Statement**
SICK PAY PURPOSES ONLY   **by the Doctor**

In confidence to
Mr/Mrs/Miss/Ms ....

(A) I examined you on the   (B) I have not examined you but, on the basis of a
                                   recent written report from -

following dates ....   Doctor ....(Name if known)

....   of ....

....
and advised you that you
should refrain from work   .... (Address)

....   I have advised you that you should refrain

from .... to ....   from work for/until ....

Diagnosis of your disorder
causing   absence   from   ....
work Doctor's remarks.

Doctor's   Date of
signature   signing

The special circumstances in which this form may be used are described in the
handbook "A guide for registered medical practitioners."

                                                                Form Med 5

PATIENT TO COMPLETE PARTICULARS ON REVERSE

Printed for BA OSD/PCMG by PADS 008984P 11/99

Figure 4.2   Form Med 5 (sample).

TO BE COMPLETED IN ALL CASES - PLEASE USE BLOCK LETTERS
If you cannot fill this form in yourself, ask someone else to do so.

Surname Mr/Mrs/Miss/Ms

First names

Present address

Postcode

	Date	Month	Year

Date of birth

National Insurance Number

Works or Clock Number
or Department

If the doctor has given you a date to resume work
date you intend to start (or
seek) work for an employer
or as a self-employed person

	Date	Month	Year
day			

For night shift
workers only

Time   am/pm
Time   am/pm

FOR STATE BENEFIT CLAIMANTS ONLY
If you wish to claim benefit, continue below. To avoid losing benefit send this form
QUICKLY to your local Social Security Office.
NOTE: To start your claim for State benefit you must use form SC1 if you are self-
employed, unemployed or non-employed OR form SSP1 if you are an employee.
For further details get leaflet FB28 (from Social Security local offices)

Full name and address
of employer (if employed)

| DECLARATION |

Remember: If you give information that is incorrect or incomplete action may be taken
against you.
I declare that because of incapacity I have not worked since the date of my last claim. I also
declare that my circumstances and those of my dependants are and have been as last
stated. (If there has been a change cross out this declaration and attach a signed and dated
statement of new facts.)
I declare that the information I have given on this form is correct and complete.
I agree that the Department of Social Security or a doctor acting on their behalf may get in
touch with my doctor so that they may give the Department of Social Security any information
which is needed to deal with this claim and any request to look at the claim again.

Sign
here ....   Date ....
If you have signed on behalf of the person
claiming tick the box.

Figure 4.2   Continued.

confirmation by another doctor. Two signatures are always necessary, and a doctor may be asked to sign in either capacity. These certificates are available from local funeral directors, and the secretary or receptionist may be asked to ensure that there are forms available when required. A fee is payable to both signatories.

Private certification

Private certificates are issued to patients for purposes outside the scope of the NHS. They are used to supply information to organisations concerning proof of illness, such as the following:

*   holiday insurance

*   sick pay and superannuation purposes

*   solicitors

*   insurance companies

*   schools.

A fee may be charged for private certificates. The BMA makes recommendations for fees, and doctors will charge according to their recommended scale.

Certificate of stillbirth

A doctor must sign a certificate of stillbirth if he or she was present at the delivery or examined the body of a stillborn child, and must give it to the person who will inform the registrar.

Birth registration

Every live birth or stillbirth must be registered within 42 days. It is the duty of either of the parents to register the birth. In the case of an illegitimate child, the duty to register the birth rests with the mother.

All certificates should either be stamped with the doctor's name, address, etc., or be printed in the case of a private certificate.

The Local Medical Officer must be notified of all births, either by the hospital or by the doctor in attendance.

Abortion certificates (termination of pregnancy)

The law in the UK allows doctors to terminate pregnancies as long as certain conditions are met:

1   two doctors must see the patient
2   they must agree that the conditions laid down in the 1967 Abortion Act have been satisfied.

Note: These conditions allow doctors to recommend termination when they feel that to continue with the pregnancy would be a hazard to either the physical or mental welfare of the pregnant woman or to any existing children of her family.

Secretaries and receptionists may be responsible for ensuring that the appropriate certification forms are available when required (*see* Figure 4.3).

Health and safety at work

The legislation relating to health and safety at work is complex, and although they are not directly responsible for workplace standards, medical secretaries and receptionists should be aware of the implications of the Health and Safety at Work etc. Act 1974 and of their personal responsibilities.

Health and Safety at Work etc. Act 1974

This Act, which was passed in 1974, is of direct relevance to individuals, whether as managers responsible for the safety of staff immediately under their control, or as a member of the team responsible for the health and safety standards in the surgery, hospital outpatient department or clinic. The Health and Safety at Work etc. Act 1974 is a criminal statute and the Health and Safety Executive (HSE) is the enforcement body. Failure to carry out any duty under the Act is an offence and can lead to prosecution.

The aim of the legislation is to provide and create workplace standards for the reduction of known hazards, provision of a safe working environment for employees and adequate training and supervision given as is necessary to ensure, so far as is reasonably practicable, the health and safety at work of employees. All employers must fulfil this obligation. The term 'reasonably practicable' may be inferred from case law and the advice of HSE inspectors.

HSE inspectors have considerable powers, and may enter premises to enforce the law. Although they do not need to ask permission before doing

---

IN CONFIDENCE   **CERTIFICATE A**

ABORTION ACT 1967

Not to be destroyed within three years of the date of operation

**Certificate to be completed before an abortion is
performed under Section 1(1) of the Act**

I, ...
(Name and qualifications of practitioner in block capitals)

of ....

....
(Full address of practitioner)

Have/have not* seen/and examined* the pregnant woman to whom this certificate relates at

....

....
(full address of place at which patient was seen or examined)

on ....

and I ....
(Name and qualifications of practitioner in block capitals)

of ....

....
(Full address of practitioner)

Have/have not* seen/and examined* the pregnant woman to whom this certificate relates at

....

....
(Full address of place at which patient was seen or examined)

on ....

We hereby certify that we are of the opinion, formed in good faith, that in the case

of ....
(Full name of pregnant woman in block capitals)

of ....

....
(Usual place of residence of pregnant woman in block capitals)

(Ring appro-priate letter(s))	A	the continuance of the pregnancy would involve risk to the life of the pregnant woman greater than if the pregnancy were terminated;
	B	the termination is necessary to prevent grave permanent injury to the physical or mental health of the pregnant woman;
	C	the pregnancy has NOT exceeded its 24th week and that the continuance of the pregnancy would involve risk, greater than if the pregnancy were terminated, of injury to the physical or mental health of the pregnant woman;
	D	the pregnancy has NOT exceeded its 24th week and that the continuance of the pregnancy would involve risk, greater than if the pregnancy were terminated, of injury to the physical or mental health of any existing child(ren) of the family of the pregnant woman;
	E	there is a substantial risk that if the child were born it would suffer from such physical or mental abnormalities as to be seriously handicapped.

**This certificate of opinion is given before the commencement of the treatment for the termination
of pregnancy to which it refers and relates to the circumstances of the pregnant woman's
individual case.**

Signed ....   **Date** ....

Signed ....   **Date** ....

* Delete as appropriate   D-IDH005329 4-94 C8000 CC38806   Form HSA1 (revised 1991)

Figure 4.3   Abortion certification form (sample).

so, they usually telephone to arrange a visit. Sanctions may be imposed upon those who have unlawfully created or permitted hazards, even where no one has suffered an accident or ill health.

Employees themselves are obliged to take reasonable care to help to meet this statutory requirement ('legal duty of care').

Duties of employers and employees

The duties arising from the Health and Safety at Work etc. Act 1974 are not difficult to apply. The legislation requires an employer (including a self-employed person, such as a GP) to provide and maintain a safe working environment, and it establishes powers and penalties to enforce this. The main aim of the Act is to make both employers and employees conscious of the need for safety in all aspects of their work.

Employers' general duties to staff

The most important duty which every employer should fulfil is 'to ensure as far as is reasonably practicable, the health, safety and welfare at work of all his employees' (Health and Safety at Work etc. Act 1974).

Written statement of safety policy

An employer should provide information, training and supervision for staff on health and safety matters. Unless there are fewer than five staff, employers must provide a statement of general policy on health and safety and ensure that it is implemented; employees should be consulted on its form and content. The written statement may be included in your employment contract. However, in a medical practice with fewer than five staff, it is not necessary to give everyone a copy, and the statement can be displayed in a public place.

Safety representatives

Safety representatives are usually appointed if an employer recognises a trade union (e.g. hospitals, health centres). They have a right to challenge the employer on all health and safety matters.

Duties to others using the hospital or surgery

An employer must ensure the safety of anyone using the premises, including patients, medical and pharmaceutical representatives, visitors, builders, tradesmen and health authority staff.

The Act requires the hospital, surgery or clinic to be run so as to ensure that all users of the premises are safe from risks of personal injury, and consideration should be given as to whether there are any potential hazards to elderly or disabled patients.

Notifying accidents and dangerous occurrences

An employer should keep a record of accidents. The HSE should be informed of certain serious accidents that befall anyone using the premises.

Employees' responsibilities

Staff are required to take reasonable care of their own health and safety on the premises, and of the safety of other users of the premises who may be affected by their actions or omissions, and are expected to co-operate with the employer in carrying out these duties. Although employees' duties technically apply while at work, it would be wise to assume that they also apply throughout the time the employees are on the premises (e.g. when preparing coffee or lunch in a staff rest-room).

Staff must not interfere with or misuse any health and safety equipment (e.g. fire exits, fire extinguishers and warning notices).

Health and safety at work – regulations

In January 1993, six new sets of health and safety at work regulations came into force. They apply to almost all types of work activity in hospitals and general practice. Like the health and safety law, they place duties on employers to protect:

*   their employees
*   others, including members of the public who may be affected by the work being done.

These new regulations are needed to implement six European Community (EC) directives on health and safety at work. At the same time, they are part of the continuing modernisation of UK law, and cover the following:

*   health and safety management (revised in 1999)
*   work equipment safety (revised in 1998)
*   manual handling of loads
*   workplace conditions

- personal protective equipment
- display-screen equipment.

Management of health and safety at work (1999)

The regulations require employers to:

- assess the risk to the health and safety of their employees and anyone else who may be affected by their work in order to identify any necessary preventive and protective measures. Employers with five or more employees should write their risk assessment down

- make arrangements for putting into practice the preventive and protective measures that follow from this risk assessment: they should cover planning, organisation control, monitoring and review (i.e. the management of health and safety). Again, any employer with five or more employees must put these arrangements in writing

- carry out health surveillance of employees when appropriate

- appoint a competent person (normally an employee) to help to devise and apply the protective steps that the risk assessment shows to be necessary

- set up emergency procedures

- give employees information about health and safety matters

- co-operate on health and safety matters with other employers sharing the same premises (e.g. other health authorities)

- make sure that employees have adequate health and safety training and are sufficiently capable at their job to avoid risk

- give whatever health and safety information temporary staff need to meet their specific needs.

These regulations also:

- place duties on all employees to follow health and safety instructions and report danger

- extend current health and safety laws which require employers to consult employees' safety representatives and provide facilities for them.

Provision and use of work equipment (1998)

These regulations pull together and tidy up various laws governing equipment used at work. These regulations:

- place general duties on all employers
- list minimum requirements for work equipment to deal with selected hazards which apply across all industries and sectors.

Generally speaking, these regulations make explicit what is already provided for elsewhere in current legislation or in good practice. Organisations that have well-chosen and well-maintained equipment need not do any more. The general duties of these regulations require organisations to:

- take into account the working conditions and hazards in the workplace when choosing equipment
- make sure that equipment is suitable for the use intended and that it is properly maintained
- give adequate information, instruction and training.

Manual handling operations (1992)

These regulations replace patchy, old-fashioned and largely ineffective legislation with a modern ergonomic approach to the problems of manual handling. They are important because the incorrect handling of loads may cause injuries, resulting in pain, time off work and even permanent disablement.

They apply to any manual handling operations which may cause injury at work. The manual handling assessment is a specific requirement under this regulation. The safety management regulations include not only lifting loads, but also lowering, pushing, pulling, carrying or moving them, whether by hand or by means of other bodily force. Again, these regulations are supported by general guidance.

There are healthcare areas where staff are at risk in this respect, such as nursing. Employers have to take four key steps.

1 Avoid hazardous manual handling operations when it is reasonably practicable to do so.

2 Assess adequately any hazardous operations that cannot be avoided.

3 Reduce the risk of injury as far as possible.

4 Review assessments when changes take place.

Workplace health, safety and welfare (1992)

These regulations tidy up much of the existing legislation, replacing some 35 pieces of old law. They are much easier to understand and make it far clearer what is expected. They cover many aspects of health, safety and welfare in the workplace, setting general requirements in four broad areas:

1   *working environment* – temperature, ventilation, lighting, room dimensions, suitability of workstations

2   *safety* – safe passage of pedestrians and vehicles, windows and skylights (safe opening, closing and cleaning), safe materials and marking for transparent doors and partitions, doors, gates and escalators (safety devices), safe doors, gates and escalators, floors, falls from heights and falling objects

3   *facilities* – toilets, washing, eating and changing facilities, clothing storage, seating, rest areas, arrangements for non-smokers and rest facilities

4   *housekeeping* – maintenance of workplace, equipment and facilities, cleanliness, and removal of waste materials.

Employers should ensure that their premises comply with these regulations.

Personal protective equipment (1992)

These regulations set out sound principles for selecting, providing, maintaining and using personal protective equipment (PPE). They are not directly relevant to medical secretaries and receptionists, so further information would be inappropriate here.

Display-screen equipment (DSE) (1992)

Unlike most of the regulations previously listed, the health and safety (display-screen equipment) regulations do not replace old legislation, but cover a new area of work activity. Working with DSE is not generally risky, but it can lead to musculoskeletal problems, eye fatigue and mental stress. Problems of this kind can be overcome by good ergonomic design of equipment, furniture, the working environment and the tasks performed.

The regulations apply to DSE where there is a regular user (i.e. an employee who habitually uses it as a significant part of normal work). They cover equipment used for the display of text, numbers and graphics, regardless of the display process used.

These regulations include the following:

- assessing DSE workstations and reducing risks which are identified

- making sure that workstations satisfy minimum requirements set for the DSE itself – keyboard, desk and chair, working environment and task design and software

- planning DSE work so that there are breaks or changes in activity

- providing information and training for DSE users.

DSE users are entitled to appropriate eye and eyesight tests, and to corrective glasses if they are needed and normal spectacles cannot be used. Again these regulations are supported by detailed guidelines which are contained in the Health and Safety Executive's *Guidance Note on DSE Work*.

The Control of Substances Hazardous to Health Regulations (COSHH) 1999

COSHH regulations set out guidelines for the control of hazardous substances to employers, who have an obligation to protect people exposed to such substances.

The regulations include virtually all substances which are hazardous to health, and clearly set out the essential measures which employers, the self-employed, and sometimes employees, have to take. Failure to comply constitutes an offence under the Health and Safety at Work etc. Act 1974. Substances hazardous to health include those labelled as:

- dangerous

- toxic

- harmful

- irritant

- corrosive.

The regulations give guidelines to employers which are based upon principles of occupational hygiene, the key duties being:

- to identify substances hazardous to health in the workplace

- to assess formally (in writing) the risk to employees from these materials

- to control adequately and monitor the risk

- to provide health surveillance where appropriate

- to provide adequate instruction and training.

Other less dangerous substances covered by the regulations include disinfectants, clinical wastes and cleaning materials.

GPs, health authorities and other healthcare employers should consider how COSHH applies to the working environment and to their employees, for example:

- the risk from biocides and sterilising agents

- the risk of staff contracting infection from biological samples and waste

- policies and specific procedures are necessary for cleaning medical equipment, and safe disposal of drugs, contaminated needles, dressings and appliances

- staff vaccination status should be reviewed.

Summary of legal aspects

This section has attempted to give an overview of the many and diverse legal aspects involving the work of medical secretaries and receptionists.

On a more personal note, information has been given to provide a basic knowledge and understanding of the legislation that influences the duties and rights of employees and employers working in organisations, large or small.

5

Health and safety in a clinical environment

Introduction

General principles of health and safety at work have already been discussed in some detail. On a practical level, how does this affect the secretary and receptionist working in a clinical environment?

The Health and Safety at Work etc. Act 1974 requires:

- *that any 'plant' in the workplace is safe* – the term 'plant' covers equipment in the work environment, including heaters, sterilisers, electric kettles, plugs and examination couches. Potential hazards include someone getting a shock from an electric kettle due to a plug being incorrectly fitted, or a patient being injured because an examination couch collapses. Occurrences such as these could lead to a charge of having unsafe plant on the premises and ensuing liability. Electrical and mechanical equipment needs to be serviced at least annually

- *that systems of work are safe* – it is important that day-to-day work systems are safe and do not lead to injury. Safe systems normally refer to policy and procedures (e.g. manual handling risk assessment and the use of gloves while handling specimens)

- *that premises are safe* – this includes floors which are uneven and/or slippery or dangerous when wet, outside steps which are uneven and/or unlit at night, and ceilings in danger of collapse, which could all be regarded as unsafe.

First aid at work

Regulations require employers to make adequate provision for their employees in case of injury or if they should become unwell at work. It is advisable, but not mandatory, to have a qualified first aider, although a doctor or a nurse could become an 'appointed person' – but there must be an appointed person available at all times. This person is to take charge of the situation should a serious injury or illness occur in the workplace and is responsible for the first-aid equipment. An 'appointed person', if not fully trained, should have attended a short course in first aid lasting a minimum of four hours, which should include the following:

- resuscitation

- control of bleeding

- treatment of the unconscious casualty.

Hazardous substances in the workplace

Control of Substances Hazardous to Health (COSHH) regulations have already been mentioned. Receptionists and secretaries should be aware of hazards arising from the handling, transport, storage and disposal of hazardous substances. Control measures must be in place to ensure that their place of work is not in breach of the law.

Clinical waste

Clinical waste is waste arising from medical practice that may provide a hazard or give offence unless it is rendered safe and inoffensive. Such waste includes human or animal tissue or excretions, drugs and medicinal products, swabs, dressings, instruments or similar substances and materials.

All staff involved in areas where clinical waste arises should be given instruction in waste handling, segregation, storage and disposal procedures and, where appropriate, the use of protective clothing.

Waste segregation

This is achieved by the use of readily identifiable colour-coded containers or plastic bags:

- *black* – normal household waste only
- *yellow* – clinical waste for incineration.

There are different categories of waste and different procedures for each category. These include the following:

- soiled surgical dressings, swabs and other contaminated waste from consulting rooms and treatment areas
- syringes, needles, cartridges and glass ampoules ('sharps'). It is dangerous to dispose of 'sharps' in yellow bags, as this is a potential cause of needlestick injuries
- laboratory waste in medical practice, including blood samples, vomit or sputum
- solid-dose medicinal products, small-volume injectables, vaccine and sera*
- urine samples.

Secretaries and receptionists will be given appropriate instructions for disposal if necessary. However, the following guidelines should be understood by all those working in medical practice.

Storage of clinical waste

Waste bags must be kept secure from unauthorised persons and entry by animals whilst awaiting collection. They must never be left outside where children may play, or where drug addicts may find used syringes and needles.

Removal of clinical waste

This is arranged on a local basis. Health authorities/health boards will advise on the availability of a collection service. Organisations providing this will arrange to supply services and arrange collection and incineration.

*All controlled drugs covered by the Misuse of Drugs Act require special procedures before they can be destroyed. Unused drugs are usually returned to the pharmacy for safe disposal.

Specimens

Handling specimens

Receptionists in general practice may find that patients leave various specimens on the reception counter unwrapped. It is the receptionist's duty to protect herself and colleagues from potential infection by handling these specimens correctly. For example, either ask the patient to place the specimen in a plastic bag, or use a pair of disposable gloves to handle the specimen. The same system could be used for handling used medicine containers, dressings, tissues, hearing aids, etc.

Transport of specimens

Specimens to be sent to the pathology laboratory by the local collection service must be clearly labelled and accompanied by pathology request forms. Specimens to be sent by post must be packaged in a rigid container with absorbent packing and sent by first-class letter post. The address of the sender should be clearly written on the outside of the package so that the post office can contact the sender if the package is damaged, in order to ascertain the risk to the handler. Specimens sent through the post must be clearly labelled 'Pathological Specimen – Handle with Care'.

Hepatitis and AIDS

Receptionists are at risk in situations where blood, semen and other body fluids of an infected person can enter the body (e.g. through an open cut). All scratches, cuts and grazes must be covered with a waterproof dressing.

When body fluid has to be mopped up, disposable plastic or latex gloves, a disposable plastic apron and paper tissues must be used *whether or not* infection is present. After use, these items must be placed in a clinical waste collection unit for incineration. Clothing may be cleaned by washing on a hot cycle. Hard surfaces and floors can be wiped/washed with a freshly prepared 10% bleach solution. Skin that has been in contact should be washed with soap and water. Mouth-to-mouth resuscitation should be carried out with a mouthpiece if one is available. Common-sense measures and good hygiene are the best ways to prevent infection.

The likelihood of staff being infected with hepatitis is considerably higher than with AIDS, as the virus survives at room temperature for a much longer duration. Hepatitis B vaccination is available to staff for protection.

Fire Precautions Act 1971

This is the Act that covers fire regulations. However, in medical practices with less than 20 employees there is no need for a fire certificate. Larger organisations (e.g. hospitals and health centres) will have regular fire drills. The local fire officer will check the provision of fire alarms, extinguishers and hoses, and that fire exits are not obstructed and signs are readily visible. The provision of emergency light supplies is also checked.

Medical practices should have their own plans and clearly defined procedures to be followed in the event of a fire. Basic guidelines would include the following:

- *prevention* – check for hazards and try to prevent a fire from occurring

- *fire alert/warning* – who will raise the alarm and dial 999? Who will evacuate the surgery? What is the system for ensuring that everyone in the building knows about the fire? How can more patients be prevented from entering?

- *evacuation* – procedures for evacuating the building. Marshall all staff and patients to one assembly point. Check that no one is missing

- *security* – people are most important. Leave behind all valuables except the appointment book, which will tell you if anyone is missing. This should be taken to the assembly point

- *informing staff and the public* – a notice should be displayed telling people what to do in the event of a fire. The notice should indicate the assembly point and the action to be taken in the event of a fire.

Clinical risk management

Although risk management is not new, its application to clinical medicine is a relatively new concept in the UK. It is a response to increasing medical litigation but, in addition to reducing the chance (or cost) of litigation, it should lead to improved patient care. In a hospital, one of the greatest areas of risk in financial terms arises from patient treatment. Clinical risk management programmes require the active involvement of senior and junior medical staff, nurses and other healthcare professionals. Clinical risk management may be categorised as follows:

- accident prevention

- damage limitation.

Accident prevention means taking steps to avoid adverse outcomes, and it includes the following:

- continuing medical education

- clinical audit

- protocols and guidelines for treatment

- the application of results from previous claims.

For example, a primary prevention step may be for a new member of staff in accident and emergency to know which facilities are immediately available and how and when to summon more experienced assistance.

Damage limitation measures either help in the investigation of a problem, or are steps taken to ensure that events or incidents are routinely investigated.

Clinical risk management is not about gathering information and form filling, but rather it is concerned with identifying and analysing the risk and then controlling the latter. Controlling the risk is the most important element, as the ultimate aim is accident prevention.

Coping with aggression and violence

Violence against NHS staff is becoming more and more of a problem. It requires action at the highest level to find a solution. The Government has promoted a campaign of zero tolerance, which aims to:

- ensure that the public are aware that violence against NHS staff is unacceptable

- reassure NHS staff that acts of violence and intimidation against them are not acceptable, and that they have taken action to combat them.

In 1998, the Government set the NHS a target of cutting acts of violence against staff by 29% by 2001, increasing to 30% by 2003. NHS trusts have published strategies to achieve these targets and to monitor their outcomes.

A requirement of the Crime and Disorder Act of 1998 is that the police and local authorities should work with organisations, including NHS trusts and health authorities, to bring in strategies to combat crime and disorder.

Dealing with aggressive callers

Receptionists and secretaries working in the field of healthcare face a number of patients and callers who are potentially violent (e.g. the mentally disturbed, the emotionally upset, or those who are suffering from the effects of drugs or alcohol).

Your organisation will no doubt have a policy for dealing with potentially violent patients. If so, it is up to you to ensure that you know what it is and what you should do. Remember that most of the patients attending your hospital or your surgery are seeking understanding, help and advice about problems which are causing them a certain amount of anxiety. They may become frustrated and aggrieved as they wait for their appointments.

As a patient becomes more upset, this can lead to aggression and the receptionist or secretary may be the focus of the latter. Always deal as quickly as possible with any patient who becomes agitated, especially if they seem to be under the influence of drugs or alcohol. Make sure that you alert the doctor or nurse to the problem as soon as possible.

If a confrontation is developing, try to defuse the situation by talking to the patient in a calm manner, and attempt to reduce their agitation. You may be able to distract the patient from their particular grievance and cool the situation.

You should be on guard to protect yourself from physical attack. If you are trying to appear relaxed and natural you may, for example, put your hands in your pockets – this will leave you defenceless to a blow. If possible, always put a physical barrier (e.g. a computer or desk) between yourself and the aggressor. Discreetly try to attract the attention of another member of staff if it seems as if the situation is going to erupt. If you have a buzzer 'alert' or panic button system, have a prearranged signal and use it.

NHS organisations are installing closed-circuit television (CCTV), which will often act as a deterrent.

Note: The best way to defend yourself from attack is to get out of the way as quickly as possible.

Coping with a personal attack

A personal attack is unlikely to occur, and if you take common-sense precautions you can reduce the risk. Unfortunately, some attacks do occur and you should give some thought to what you would do if you were a victim.

Always remember that personal safety should come before property. Is it worth being injured for the sake of a prescription or some tablets? The police would prefer you uninjured and in a position to give them an accurate description of the attacker.

It is worth considering what you would be prepared to do in self-defence should you be attacked. If other people are nearby, then you must shout to attract their attention. Only you can decide whether to fight back. A woman has the right to defensive action using reasonable force in the case of an attack – for example, by kicking, scratching or by the use of items which are accepted as normally being carried, such as:

* hair-spray

* bunch of keys

* umbrella

* personal attack alarm.

However, it must be pointed out that legally you may not carry offensive weapons.

If you are sexually assaulted or raped, it is important that you contact the police immediately – both for your own sake and for the safety of others. Always bear in mind:

* however difficult or unpleasant the thought, resist the urge to wash or change your clothing – you could be removing important evidence

* do not drink alcohol or take any drugs that might prevent you from giving a clear account of what has happened

* try to remember as much as possible about your attacker.

The police will deal with you with care, understanding and complete confidentiality.

General security and safety in the surgery or hospital

* Challenge all suspicious individuals.

* Do not be taken in by so-called workmen or officials; if they are genuine, they will not mind having their identity checked.

* Keep all valuables and prescription pads out of sight.

* Ensure that petty cash is secured in a locked tin, and kept inside a locked drawer.

* Ensure that consulting and treatment rooms are locked when not in use.

* If you have an identity badge, always wear it.

* Equipment should be security marked.

* Always keep your valuables with you, or lock them away.

Travelling to and from work or whenever you are out and about

You should always be alert to potential danger when travelling by car, public transport or on foot. Remember the following points.

- Think ahead. Get into a safe routine and always use it.
- Avoid walking home late at night.
- Walk purposefully. Do *not* accept lifts.
- When travelling by car, do not give lifts to strangers.
- On public transport, sit near the guard, driver or other women passengers.
- Only use a reputable taxi-cab firm. Ask the cab company for the driver's name and call sign.
- In the event of your car breaking down, while you are waiting for help make sure that you keep the doors and windows locked and sit in the passenger seat so that you do not appear to be alone.
- Avoid using multi-storey car parks if possible.
- Carry a torch with you if you are travelling after dark.

Safety at the end of a surgery or clinic session

Always check that the premises are secure before you leave, and look outside to make sure that no one is lurking. If you see someone prowling or hanging around, stay inside and let someone know. If necessary, contact the police. If you are usually collected by car, wait until it arrives before going out. If you are travelling by public transport and are alone, do not leave so early that you have to wait a long time for the bus or train.

Finally, your local crime prevention officer attached to your nearest police station will be willing to talk to you and your colleagues about coping with aggression and violence, and give practical help and advice to women about their personal safety.

6

Practical reception skills in general practice

Introduction

Every receptionist is gifted in some way, for example in dealing kindly with people, having patience, a pleasant speaking voice, etc. In addition to these natural gifts, everyone can acquire skills to help them to do their job better. The most important skill areas are those of communication and organisation, which are covered in other areas of this text. However, there are some skills which are unique to a receptionist in general practice.

All approaches to the receptionist are by patients, or their relatives, who believe that they have a need. They cannot see 'behind the scenes' in the surgery or have any real understanding of the pressures on doctors and receptionists. Receptionists must always bear in mind the perceived need of the patient, no matter how insignificant it may seem from the surgery perspective. Patients are concerned about either their own state of health or that of a family member. It is very important, therefore, that the skills of recognising how patients are feeling and dealing sensitively with them are used constantly. Non-verbal communication and related issues are covered in Chapter 2.

The person responsible for controlling the flow of patients into a number of doctors consulting at the same time needs to have a good system, to concentrate and remain alert. If other members are fully co-operative in matters such as ensuring that the appointments book or surgery lists are clearly written, or appropriately 'marking off' a patient as arriving, or having been sent into the doctor, then the task is made simpler. However, the person controlling the surgery flow tends to be the one to whom everyone turns with queries. Where are Mrs A's results? Where are the notes for child B? Do I need to do a claim form for child health surveillance? How many extras are there? When will Dr C be free to see the rep? And so on. If telephone answering is also part of the picture, it can be very difficult to keep on top of who is where, and what needs to be dealt with next.

Smooth surgery flow is made easier if the preparation for surgeries has been carried out properly. Where an appointment system is used, it is sensible to take out all the medical records well before the start of surgery, and check that all of the test results and hospital letters relating to these records have been filed. It can also help the practice finances if stickers are used on the records to indicate that smears are due or pill forms need to be signed, which the receptionist can then act upon by drawing the doctor's attention with a note, or completing a claim ready for signature.

As patients leave the consulting-room, follow-up appointments need to be arranged and appropriate advice given about requirements for some health promotion clinics (e.g. to bring a urine sample). Maintaining neat work areas during consulting times makes tidying at the end of surgery considerably easier. However, even if it is not possible to keep tidy at the busiest times, it is important that quieter times are used to the full to return working areas to order, file medical records, and check that doctors' rooms have been tidied and that stocks of disposables topped up.

Telephone answering can be an especially difficult task for the doctor's receptionist. Any incoming call may be about a patient who is bleeding, appearing to have a heart attack, or experiencing some other medical crisis with a child. Therefore the procedure for dealing with emergencies must be clear and the telephone must never be left to ring for an indefinite period. The telephone must be answered in preference to dealing with a patient standing at the reception desk. However, it is also essential that any patient at the desk is acknowledged with a smile, so that they know they will be dealt with when you are free.

The receptionist is also required to be a fount of all knowledge. For example, the following can be helpful in finding and giving out appropriate information efficiently:

- keeping telephone directories of often used numbers, or hospital internal directories, along with other service information sources

- a list of subjects of leaflets kept available for patients in the waiting-room and brief notes on developments in trends in health promotion

- a list giving addresses and telephone numbers of self-help groups and voluntary organisations

- awareness of changes to surgeries and clinics, and changes in local hospital, community and social services.

It is especially important that the receptionist knows the limits of her own authority (i.e. when and to whom to refer for advice).

The receptionist is also responsible for keeping an eye on the waiting-area to:

- make sure that the patients who are obviously unwell are not troubled by unduly active children

- generally keep a watchful eye on the waiting-area, and note if any patients appear to be unduly distressed or extremely unwell

- maintain a pleasant ambience by ensuring adequate ventilation or heat

- tidy the waiting-area of toys, magazines and leaflets at the end of each surgery or clinic.

Thankfully, it will rarely be necessary to clean up whilst patients are waiting (e.g. if a patient is literally sick in the waiting-area or treads something unpleasant-smelling from the pavement into the surgery!).

Keeping the doctors happy is yet another set of tasks for the receptionist. Most of the time this will entail keeping the surgery flow steady, not allowing too many interruptions in consultations, providing tea or coffee at the right times, and making sure that records, results, letters and other essentials are all available when required. Not too much to ask!

Individually controlling surgery flow, answering the telephone, dealing with patients at the desk, and keeping the doctor happy are not too difficult to achieve as separate items, but in the real world of the reception office there is rarely the opportunity to concentrate on one task at a time. The skill is in being able to readjust priorities constantly, without forgetting the ones that slip to the bottom of the mental pile.

Dividing up the duties so that, for instance, one person controls surgery flow, another concentrates on answering the telephone, and another does repeat prescriptions and perhaps deals with queries, can go some way towards reducing the pressure. However, it is also impossible to adhere rigidly to such a plan. It is essential that receptionists work in a team, not only keeping on top of what they are supposed to be doing, but also having their eyes open to see when a colleague needs help, and being able to adjust their own priorities to step into the breach.

Various tools, such as log books, message books, having good systems in place, having clear procedures for dealing with routine issues, and knowing whom to turn to with queries, all help. However, the ability to juggle ten priorities at one time is both an art and a gift. Being self-controlled, planning work, and being as efficient about it as possible means that anyone with a degree of intelligence, who wants to, can achieve a certain degree of competency. However, there will always be some people who enjoy this kind of pressure (only feeling the strain sometimes) and some to whom it is a strain all the time.

First impressions

First impressions count. A receptionist will often be the patient's initial point of contact with the organisation, and they will make assumptions (positive or negative) about the treatment that they are likely to receive from that first point.

Record keeping and general administration

In any business it is essential to keep records. For example, where a receptionist may be delegated the task of keeping control of stocks of forms and stationery, or petty cash, it is essential that adequate documentation is maintained. Alternatively, a receptionist is likely to pass messages to a variety of people in the course of a working day. Keeping a record of messages ensures that not only does the right message get passed, but the person who took the message, the person who received it, and when, can all be substantiated.

Written communication

Although technology is moving on apace, there is still the need for handwritten communication – messages and notes from one person to another. It is obvious that any handwritten communication should be legible, but often in haste it is easy to forget this, and to fail to ensure that any other person can read a scrawled message, entry in an appointment book or list of names, etc.

Messages

Some offices have preprinted message forms which prompt message takers to collect all of the necessary information as they go. Another option is to use a message book with columns drawn up, so that it is easy to check whether a message has been received. It is important not only that there should be adequate systems for communicating messages, but also that responsibility is taken to ensure that the systems work properly.

Message-boards

Dry-wipe white-boards are extremely useful for putting up short-term reminders and messages, provided that one person is delegated responsibility for wiping off messages as soon as they become redundant!

Letters and memos

Receptionists may be required to send out letters and memos. As a general rule these are likely to be routine (standard) documents, where a master copy is used to generate photocopies, into which names and addresses, dates and data can be inserted by hand. However, technology has made it possible for receptionists with little or no formal training in secretarial or wordprocessing skills to generate printed letters from the computer. It is vital to remember that the image of the practice/hospital is presented via written communication, and therefore it is vital that presentation standards are met. There are conventions about letter layout (e.g. whether commas are used at the end of every line in an address or how many spaces are left between the end of a letter and 'Yours sincerely'). Where training is not given in these details, a poor impression will be conveyed to anyone who expects normal conventions to be observed. Therefore the setting of practice standards is a valuable guide to ensure that everyone produces written communication to the same standard.

Organisation

Systems and organisation are essential to the smooth running of a reception area. Some people are blessed with a natural ability to be organised. Those who are not need to apply far more self-discipline in order to initiate and maintain systems. Everyone needs to know what is expected of whom, using what, and by when.

Similarly, individuals need to be organised in their use of time. The receptionist who retains control of the tasks to be completed avoids personal stress. Too much stress will inevitably lead to mistakes, poor handling of patients, and a general deterioration in standards of service.

Box 6.1

Take time out to:

1   make a list of the tasks you perform every day, every week, and once a month:

  - make a week plan

  - block off the times on the week plan when you have no option but to be 'demand driven' (e.g. on reception desk for a busy surgery/clinic)

  - fit other tasks around these blocks at the optimum time

2   make a 'to do' list

  - break down large items into small stages

  - realistically allocate items from your 'to do' list into your working week

3   discuss your findings with your supervisor so that any queries regarding priorities can be resolved to their satisfaction.

Using the simple example of stocks of forms, unless there is a system for ensuring that stocks are maintained, there is every likelihood that either one day stores will run out, or that scarce storage space will be taken up by unnecessarily large supplies.

Since there are many supplies needed, it is helpful if a system is set up and maintained with the same degree of commitment from everyone.

Initial skill is needed to think through the best and simplest way of organising any particular aspect of reception. After that, discipline and commitment from all team members are essential to maintain the system.

Maintaining the office and reception areas

In order to ensure the comfort and well-being of patients, relatives and other visitors, an effort needs to be made to keep the public areas tidy and smart. This must be a priority, because untidiness can be a hazard and gives a general impression of sloppiness.

Ensure that:

- the area is kept tidy and free from hazards. Some visitors are likely to have visual or physical disabilities

- hazards are reported promptly and immediate action is taken to minimise the danger
- fire exits are clearly indicated and kept unobstructed
- notices and information leaflets are kept up to date, and are clearly and neatly displayed
- an up-to-date supply of magazines, etc. is available for visitors to read.

Mail

Mail should be correctly sorted and date stamped on receipt. Any enclosures should be securely attached and missing items reported promptly. The mail should then be passed to the appropriate person for action.

When sending out mail, check that names and addresses are correct and clearly legible. Envelopes and parcels should be securely sealed. All of the mail you deal with should be handled promptly, as it relates to patients' health and any delay could be dangerous.

If you are suspicious of any mail received, local security arrangements should be followed. Check with your manager if you are unfamiliar with these.

It is appreciated that, for example, in some medical practices the receptionist or secretary may not be involved in handling or dealing with mail.

Stock control

The purpose of a stock control system is to keep track of such items as stationery, computer hardware, drugs, dressings, linen, sundry equipment, etc. that the practice owns. A stock control system is necessary to avoid two pitfalls:

1 *having too much stock* – money that is tied up in stock cannot be used for any other purpose, and if the stock is perishable or becomes obsolete as time passes, it may be difficult to recover this money in full

2 *having too little stock* – if essential items are scarce, patients may face long delays or inconvenience.

The ideal situation, and the one that a good stock control system aims to produce, is to have adequate stock on hand – neither too much nor too little.

Stock control also acts as a deterrent to wastage and pilfering. A good system will show when losses are occurring, and the knowledge of this may deter pilferers. It should also highlight the points at which losses are likely to occur from other causes.

Records of stock levels are obviously essential to any large-scale control system. The records may be on index cards, or a computerised stock control system may be in operation. Goods are stored until they are needed, and are released by the storekeeper only when he or she is presented with a duly authorised document, such as a requisition note.

Petty cash

Small amounts of expenditure for goods or services are usually paid for out of petty cash since the amounts are too small to be paid by cheque (e.g. stamps, milk bills, small stationery items). Secretarial or clerical staff may be responsible for controlling petty cash, and the system most commonly used is known as the *imprest* system.

The imprest amount is drawn from the account each week or month, through the main cash-book. The sum is estimated to cover all small expenses throughout the agreed period, and is referred to as the 'imprest' or 'float'. The petty cash is kept in a locked cash-box. During the month, payments are made from the imprest, and all expenditure must be covered by a petty cash voucher or a receipt. The voucher should be signed by the person receiving the money. The vouchers and receipts should be numbered and filed for purposes of audit.

A separate petty cash-book is maintained which analyses the expenditure, and at the end of the month a sum of money is drawn by cheque to restore the amount of the imprest to the original sum.

Helping to maintain a safe environment

Health and safety at work legislation is intended to safeguard all employees, patients and visitors to the workplace. Individual employees are required to ensure that they do not endanger their own health or safety, or that of their colleagues, patients or visitors. Potentially dangerous situations and unknown or potentially hazardous substances must be treated with the utmost care.

The legislation is detailed and complex. At the minimum, all staff must ensure that:

* there are no trailing wires
* filing-cabinet drawers are kept closed

- chairs and other obstacles do not block walkways or fire escapes

- fire extinguishers and exits are clearly indicated

- any known hazards are marked clearly and problems reported to the appropriate manager

- visitors are informed of any known hazards

- potentially violent situations are defused as far as is possible

- care is taken when handling specimens, especially with regard to spillages, and hands are washed after undertaking this task.

Coping with aggression and violence

Communication is often the key when dealing with conflict of this kind. Good communication can play a vital part in defusing potentially difficult situations or avoiding them altogether, but equally, poor communication can increase levels of frustration and anger which then erupt in violence (*see* Chapter 5). We have to consider carefully what messages our words and movements are conveying. Are they contradictory? We can tell when someone is saying one thing but means something quite different. Perhaps it is someone we know well, and we can therefore judge their statements on the basis of what we know of them, but it is equally likely that they are strangers, and the truth is conveyed by their stance, facial movements, etc. (*see* Chapter 2).

Procedures manuals

Many organisations are using Standard Operating Procedures (SOPs) as part of the implementation of BS5750. These SOPs state who does what, how they should do it, and how often, etc.

Within reception offices there may not be the need to have SOPs for every activity or task, but a manual of key procedures may be helpful. The administrative processes of stock control and petty cash are two examples which should be documented in a specific procedure. The procedure document may be just one side of A4 paper with the vital information summarised in a table, but it should include details of who is responsible, what steps are taken, how frequently, and any special notes. Filing these procedure sheets into a looseleaf folder allows additional procedures to be added or existing procedures to be updated whenever necessary. Apart from encouraging a uniform approach to performing tasks, these written procedures form a useful resource, especially for new staff who may have been told how to do something, but have forgotten or need to clarify the details.

Information technology (IT)

Practices still vary enormously in their modes of working, size, number of staff, equipment available, and capability of using their technology.

Computers

Where a practice has the patient database on computer, the advantages include:

- logging and generation of repeat prescriptions
- checking registration status
- checking smears, and other screening status
- checking health promotion data
- receiving email
- making appointments
- checking immunisation data and records, etc.
- receiving information from hospitals, health authorities and trusts.

If this is linked into an appointments system, the difficulties of manual appointment books (e.g. illegible writing, pages messy with cancellations, two people not being able to use the book at the same time, handwritten surgery lists for pulling out records) are all circumvented.

The major disadvantage is when the system 'goes down'. All of this increased efficiency then disappears, and returning to manual methods, no matter how temporarily, results in unavoidable delays and disruption.

Reference is made to IT for written communication in Chapter 10. Suffice it to say here that staff who could only ever write letters are now able to use wordprocessing to generate mailmerged letters, or to produce their own letters to patients with very little training. Spreadsheets can be used either to collect data (for display in tables, graphs and pie charts) or to present doctor and staff rotas.

Desktop publishing software can be used to generate leaflets, posters and handouts. Technology saves time for some tasks, while for others it does not save time, but it does make it possible to produce professional-looking documents (e.g. rota charts, posters).

For those who enjoy using the computer, it is essential that the latter does not become an obstacle between the patient and the receptionist. It is as rude to continue to type away absorbed by the machine as it is to continue to talk to a colleague or take a telephone call without acknowledging the presence of a patient.

The advantages of technology to receptionists include:

- ease of presenting professional standard documents, and speed of finding, generating and transmitting information
- efficiency in dealing with issues.

The major disadvantages to receptionists include:

- reliance on the electronics, so that if the computer 'goes down', everything has to go on hold
- the danger of losing the personal touch.

Fax

The fax machine has the following important uses in general practice:

- return of urgent blood results
- notification of discharge from maternity wards
- passing on complex information
- making claims to health authorities/health boards with regard to patient registration, etc.

In general, the advantages and disadvantages to the receptionist of using the fax machine may be summarised as follows.

Box 6.2

ADVANTAGES	*DISADVANTAGES*
Cheaper than using the telephone (if it takes less time than to say it)	Breach of confidentiality if fax goes to the wrong address
Much quicker than the post	Fax paper may fade with time, so it is important to either photocopy or file the original

---

Modern fax machines which use plain paper do not have the problem of fading print.

The Internet is a world-wide system of information technology networks, providing a global, on-line computer network that connects governments, universities, organisations and many other networks and users. The service provides:

- access to information
- on-line conversations
- information exchange
- conferences
- electronic mail.

It also has the ability to access remote computers and send and retrieve files. It began in 1984 and is now estimated to have over 50 million users, with an estimated one million new users joining each month.

Electronic mail

Electronic mail (email) is a telecommunications system that enables the users of a computer network to send messages to other users throughout the world. Telephone wires are necessary to send the signals from terminal to terminal. Email subscribers may send messages by computer by 'dropping' the communication into a central computer's memory bank by means of a modem. The recipient 'collects' the communication by means of an individual password and access-logging to safeguard against unauthorised user access to the system. Figure 6.1 shows the basic structure of an electronic mail system.

Although many GPs still continue to request investigations on pathology request forms, with results sent back to the practice on paper,

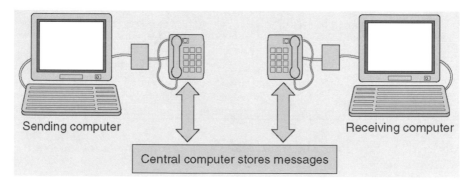

Sending computer   Receiving computer

Central computer stores messages

Figure 6.1 The basic structure of an electronic mail system. A message is sent via a telephone line and stored in a central computer. The message remains there until the recipient calls up the central computer and collects the message.

email is increasingly being used by GPs to receive electronically the results of pathological tests initiated by the practice. The way in which electronic results are used will depend on both the procedures and protocols within the practice and the features of the GP system linking with the hospital laboratory. The main benefits of laboratory links include:

- a significant reduction in the need for GPs or administrative staff to telephone the laboratory for results

- releasing administrative staff time through not having to type in test results

- the patients are impressed!

Photocopying

The photocopier is a great time saver. However, lack of training in office standards and procedures can result in poor-quality work and failure to maintain the equipment properly. Good-quality originals are essential for producing fine-quality copies. A ring binder can be kept near to the photocopier with photocopy originals in clear plastic wallets. (Yellow highlighter pen does not show up on photocopies, so use one to write 'original' to ensure that the original is easily identifiable and does not get circulated by mistake.)

Costs can be kept down by reducing the number of poor-quality copies by such simple measures as:

- collecting a folder of good-quality 'originals'

- ensuring that the original does not get used

- placing the original carefully, so that copies do not come out even slightly skewed

- buying appropriate cleaners

- keeping the platen (the glass panel on to which copies are placed) clean

- never putting documents with wet correction fluid on to the platen

- delegating someone to be responsible for replacing the toner and keeping the copier clean.

The effect of technology on staff is to make their lives a lot easier in some ways, and to make aspects of work available to them for personal development. The disadvantage for people who are afraid of technology is that they may get left behind and their value falls because they cannot take an equal share in routine workloads.

A receptionist is now required to have a wide range of skills. Apart from dealing with people on the telephone and face to face, retrieving and filing medical records and filing away letters and reports, the receptionist generally needs to have keyboard skills and a willingness to learn how to use the latest technology.

Appointment systems in general practice

The role that the medical receptionist plays is crucial to the successful running of an appointment system. Nearly every patient who sees the doctor makes his or her first contact through the receptionist. The receptionist channels patients into the appointment system and runs the system once the surgery has started.

The receptionist has to calm the agitated patient, explain and cope with doctors' absences on emergencies, and translate unstreamed demand into a rational framework.

It is important to run an appointment system as effectively as possible, for both the doctor's and the patient's sake – even a few dissatisfied patients can very quickly lead to an unhappy practice. A well-run system reflects the general efficiency of the practice, and puts less strain on GPs and their receptionists.

An efficient appointment system should benefit both doctor and patient.

Benefits to doctors include:

- effective organisation of workload

- more efficient management of time

- it limits the number of patients seen in one session

- patients' records are left on doctors' desks in advance of the surgery session

- less waiting-room space is required

- the duration of the consultation can be varied according to predetermined need.

Benefits to patients include:

- being able to plan their day

- they should not have to wait a long time to see the doctor

- there are fewer people in the waiting-room, so less likelihood of cross-infection.

The perfect appointment system is neither so rigid that it excludes emergencies, nor so chaotic that it keeps those who have made appointments waiting for an excessive length of time. The number of patients booked for each surgery session should bear a close relationship to the speed at which the doctor works.

Patient dissatisfaction arises from being unable to get an appointment without delay. Appointment systems should therefore be flexible to allow those patients with urgent problems to see their doctor very quickly.

The terms 'urgent' and 'emergency' are both subjective and emotive terms, and perhaps receptionists should be encouraged to delete them from their vocabulary! They could be replaced with 'will it wait until tomorrow?'. However, your practice will have its own procedures for dealing with such requests from patients.

Types of appointment system

Times of booking for patients can be arranged in various ways, and each practice or doctor will decide which system suits them best.

Whatever system is used, it is essential for the frequency of appointments to match the doctor's consultation rate, and for sufficient time to be left for patients who need to be seen and fitted in at short notice.

Your surgery may use one or a combination of the following types of booking:

* sequential booking

* block-release booking

* limited block booking.

All of these systems have the flexibility for patients to be seen quickly if necessary. There are several ways to deal with 'extras' to be seen despite a full appointments book:

* they can be fitted in between booked appointments

* provision can be made for patients with urgent problems to be seen after the booked surgery

* one doctor in the practice, on a rotating basis, can act as 'mopper-up' and see the extras instead of carrying out a booked surgery

* block-release booking allows 'holes' to be left in the appointments book which cannot be filled until the beginning of the day on which they are entered.

Electronic appointments

Appointments both to see the general practitioner and to see the nurse, phlebotomist, etc. are in many medical practices made by the receptionist using the computer. This allows speedy access to all booked appointments and highlights any free spaces which may be available. Hard copies can be printed off as a back-up, but doctors and nurses have access to computers and can check their own booked patients.

In addition, in some authorities it is possible to make an appointment directly for a patient consultation with a consultant at the local hospital by linking straight into their system.

Whichever method your practice uses, it is essential that the receptionist knows exactly what to do.

Follow-up after missed appointments

Patients who fail to keep their appointments for cervical cytology and immunisations will either be sent a letter or telephoned with a further appointment. If patients do not attend, doctors may not achieve their targets for cervical cytology and child immunisation.

The medical records of non-attendees for routine appointments may be marked 'DNA' or 'did not attend', and this information may also be entered on the practice computer. However, this procedure may vary according to practice protocol.

If the doctor has given the patient advice about follow-up appointments, tests, etc., it is important to check their understanding of the instructions given. They may need to be given a letter or an appointment card with the details of their next appointment. If a patient seems to be confused about what has been said, it is doubly important to encourage them to wait and have a word with the doctor or nurse before they leave. The patient may need to be directed to the correct place for any tests which are necessary. After the appointment, the notes will go to the secretary for any letters that are needed.

Many practices are now using a fully computerised appointments system to provide a more effective method of making appointments for their patients, and to replace the appointments book which can only be used by one receptionist at a time. A major benefit to the practice is that appointments can be made by as many reception staff as there are terminals.

Medical records

A medical record is the history of a patient's treatment as an outpatient, inpatient or both. The record is vital because it provides a means of communication between doctors, nurses and other members of the care team about investigations, diagnosis, observations, treatment prescribed and progress. It acts as a reminder, and can be used as an educational instrument for trainees, for research, for informing medical negligence cases and other legal purposes, and for gathering statistics such as those that are needed for planning future services.

Records contain much confidential information, and all those with access to them have a legal responsibility to maintain confidentiality. Computerised records present a particular challenge to confidentiality. This is examined in more detail in Chapter 7.

Two recent Acts of Parliament allow individuals access to their medical information. The Access to Medical Reports Act 1988 gives an individual in England, Wales or Scotland the right to see medical reports prepared for insurance or employment purposes. The Access to Personal Files and Medical Reports Order 1991 for Northern Ireland affords similar rights there. The Access to Health Records Act 1990, which applies in England, Wales and Scotland, establishes an individual's right of access to their own medical records. In certain circumstances, access can be granted to other individuals. The Act also provides for the correction of inaccurate information. Access can be refused in certain cases if, in the opinion of the record holder, disclosure would cause serious harm to the patient (*see* Chapter 4).

Medical records were standardised when the NHS began to provide some uniformity between hospitals, although some local variation still exists.

In the UK, the medical records held by general practitioners are unique: they follow patients throughout their lives from the cradle to the grave. Medical records show patients' names, demographic details, and information about previous illnesses and significant episodes in the lives of their subjects, unlike hospital records, which often only cover a specific episode of hospital attendance (e.g. for appendectomy or hysterectomy).

The purpose of the medical record

The basic function of the medical record can best be described as an *aide-mémoire* (*see* Figure 6.2).

- It gives a method of recording events in a person's life. It traces from birth the record of a patient's illnesses, treatments, investigations and other significant events.

- It is a channel of communication. The GP writes in the medical record, giving details of his or her findings, treatment and diagnosis of a patient's condition. This becomes a permanent record and communicates that information to those individuals who have the right of access (e.g. another partner in the practice, the practice nurse), or to another doctor at a later date.

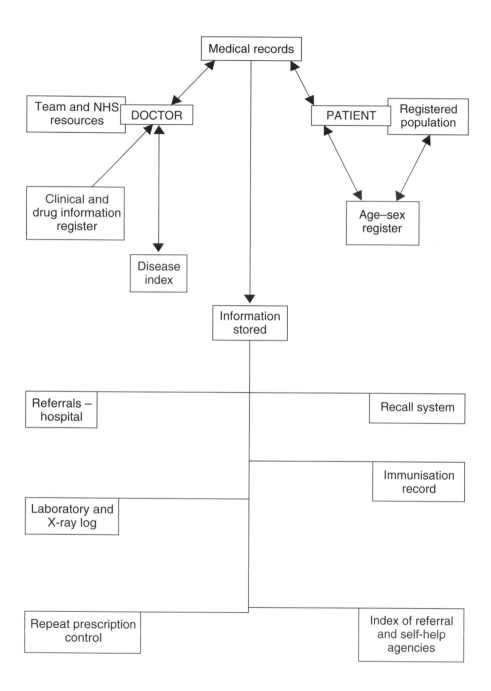

Figure 6.2   A model of the medical record information system.

- It acts as a record of outside health contacts. When the patient attends a hospital outpatient department, or has an investigation, information is provided, and if it is correctly filled in, the patient's record contributes to the total knowledge about the patient.

- It provides a record of all treatment and all of the drugs given during a patient's lifetime.

- It is a medico-legal record. If a medical or legal problem arises at any time, the patient's medical records will be required to support any action taken.

Box 6.3 The four main functions of medical records

1   A permanent record of significant events

2   A medico-legal record

3   A file for hospital and laboratory reports and letters

4   An *aide-mémoire*

Thus it is vital that medical records are kept securely and the information contained therein is stored in an orderly, systematic way. This can be achieved by:

- ensuring that all of the continuation sheets are arranged in chronological order, hopefully starting from birth, and fixing them in a permanent way (e.g. with a treasury tag), so that new continuation cards can be easily added

- keeping hospital records, copies of GPs' letters and any other correspondence in chronological order and fastened together

- dealing with the results of any investigations in the same way

- keeping a summary sheet on which the major and significant diseases or allergies are entered. This should be kept in the front of the medical record envelope (MRE)

- keeping prescription summary cards, which are also useful as a permanent, easily seen record of all drugs prescribed

- there are many other forms of record card that can be used for specific purposes, such as the child immunisation card, repeat prescription summary, obstetric record, contraceptive record, etc.

Medical receptionists and secretaries should not discard anything from a medical record envelope without the doctor's permission.

Storage of medical records

There are different ways of grouping medical records and different types of records. The most commonly used record is the small-size medical record envelope (7 × 5.5 inches) or the A4-size folder.

Some practices separate male and female records, but the majority file them together. There may be occasions when families are filed together in an A4 family folder. Every practice has its own system, but there are three main methods of storage:

1   *lateral* shelving, where records are placed side by side on shelves in alphabetical order, with alphabetical guides
2   *vertical* filing in multi-drawer cabinets, which should have alphabetical guides on the outside of the drawers
3   *carousel* or rotary filing cabinets.

A tracer or marker card should always be inserted whenever a file is pulled, and removed once the medical record is back in place. The receptionist or secretary should always check to see whether a new continuation sheet is required for doctors to record their findings.

Whatever system of filing is used in the practice, accurate filing is essential. It should be possible to pull and refile records quickly and accurately.

Confidentiality of medical records

The medical record itself has a statement at the bottom saying that it is the property of the Department of Health. However, the protection of the contents for purposes of confidentiality is the responsibility of the doctor and practice staff. Secretaries and receptionists must adhere to the rules of the practice established by the doctor with regard to who may access the information contained in the records.

Practice staff must never divulge any information contained in medical records, and great care must be taken to ensure their safe custody. Remember that many people call into the practice and may be able to see over the reception counter and read things upside down. Cleaners and maintenance staff may come into the practice when letters and other confidential information have been left lying around.

There are certain legal issues pertaining to access to medical records and data protection. These are explained fully in Chapter 4.

Much information about patients, their medical history, investigations, prescribing records, etc., is now stored on computer, but the principles of confidentiality still apply.

The medical record and information systems in general practice

The medical record is an important part of the overall information system for general practice. The record serves the needs of:

- preventive medicine

- at-risk groups of patients

- quality control measures – patient recall, performance review

- practice planning – administration and finance

- education – doctors, staff, trainees and patients

- research.

The age–sex register

The practice population can be well served by an age–sex register, which may be either a manual system or computerised, to help to identify patients at risk.

An age–sex register can be used for:

- child health surveillance

- child immunisation uptake

- cervical cytology uptake

- geriatric screening (patients over 75 years of age)

- hypertensive, diabetic and asthmatic patient screening (at-risk and chronic disease groups)

- health promotion

- an age–sex profile of the practice.

Disease or diagnostic index

Once again the system of identification of patients who have certain diseases may be either maintained manually or stored as computer data. In its simplest form in a manual system, the notes can be colour-tagged according to the system established by the Royal College of General Practitioners, which has identified eight disease groups. For example:

- red – sensitivities

- brown – diabetes

- yellow – epilepsy

- green – tuberculosis
- blue – hypertension
- white – long-term maintenance' therapy
- black – attempted suicide
- black and white chequered – measles.

The presence of a coloured tag means that the disorder is or has been present. However, the absence of a tag can never imply the absence of such a disorder.

The medical records of deceased patients can either be sent back immediately to the health authority, or await their request for return of medical records. However, this procedure may change in the near future, as many medical practices are directly linked to health authorities by computer, and such procedures can be carried out by computerised systems.

Summary

Information technology is influencing and changing many of the systems that have been used in general practice for many years. This is a time of great change, and receptionists may feel threatened by the pace at which technology is advancing. Many practices are striving to achieve a 'paperless' practice, and patients' medical records are already being stored in computer systems. Over the next few years there will be many more changes in the way in which general medical practice is run. It is an exciting and challenging time for all involved.

The hospital service

The patient's route through the hospital

The process begins with a visit by the patient either to their GP, or to an accident and emergency (A&E) department, or to one of the few direct-access services offered by some hospitals (e.g. walk-in clinics for genitourinary medicine). A GP visit results in a referral, leading to an outpatient appointment, a place on a waiting-list, attendance at a pre-assessment clinic and then admission. A direct visit to the hospital may result in a waiting-list place or even immediate admission, with the GP being informed afterwards. Alternatively, a GP refers the patient via electronic booking for day surgery (e.g. hernia repair), assesses the patient using the hospital protocol, and then books them directly on to the hospital day-surgery list. Otherwise, in some hospitals a system is in place whereby at the time of the outpatient appointment an admission date is agreed between the patient and the consultant, a pre-assessment is carried out at the clinic and the patient is admitted to hospital. This excludes the period of uncertainty while the patient is on a 'waiting-list'. Once in the hospital, the patient may be treated as an inpatient or as a day case, with access as necessary to diagnostic services, operating theatres or treatment departments.

On discharge, a summary of treatment given and follow-up needed is given to the patient's GP. Community support may be arranged, and follow-up clinic appointments may take place either in the GP's surgery or back at the hospital itself, before the patient is fully discharged (*see* Figure 7.1).

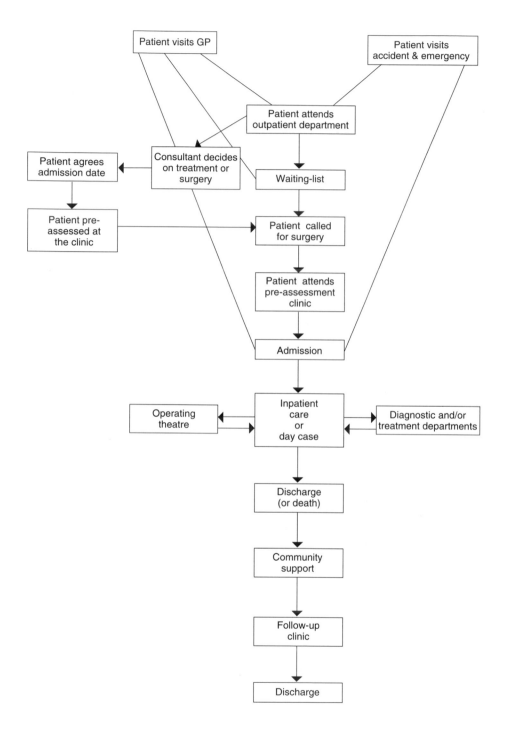

Figure 7.1   The patient's route through the hospital.

Outpatient appointments

A referral letter or specially designed referral form is sent by the GP to the appropriate consultant with an outline of the patient's condition. In exceptional circumstances a telephone referral can be made. The consultant decides how urgent the case is, and when the patient should be seen. A letter or form is then sent to the patient with details of the appointment.

If a patient has failed to turn up for a hospital appointment, this is drawn to the attention of the consultant, who decides whether another appointment should be sent or whether the GP should be informed first.

Outpatient appointments may be made centrally, or in each department, or in a mixture of both. In many hospitals the system is computerised. Each consultant generally decides how appointments are made (whether in blocks or singly), the amount of time allocated to each patient, and how many new patients and how many follow-up patients are to be booked in each clinic. New pilot systems in which patients are being given a confirmed admission date at the time of their consultation have shown that fewer patients are non-attenders, thus resulting in more efficient use of theatre time.

Referrals need not always be from a GP, but can be from the hospital's own A&E department, from another clinic, transferred from another consultant during or after treatment, or from another hospital.

On-line booking

An on-line appointment booking system has been piloted which enables GPs to book patients directly into specific consultant clinics. The 'RAPPORT' (rapid access project program for outpatient review and treatment) system enhances existing appointment booking systems. It provides a 'seamless' link between the hospital and general practitioners via the GP 'LINKS' system, giving direct access to outpatient clinics and day-case clinics.

Using the RAPPORT system, patients who do not necessarily need to see a consultant (e.g. for a hernia repair) may be booked directly by their GP for surgery, with full details of the GP's examination being mailed to the consultant (*see* Chapter 10 on using information technology).

Preparing for clinics

When preparing for a clinic, the first task is to ensure that the patient's notes are ready for doctors to refer to during the consultation. The importance of this cannot be over-emphasised, since missing or incomplete notes will result in serious difficulties for the doctor and delays for the patient. It is sensible to allow as much time as possible.

Clinic lists will be available from the appointment book or computerised patient administration system, showing all those due to attend. Case notes are then retrieved or 'pulled', double-checking for the right patient using not only their name but also their date of birth and hospital or NHS number. Checks are made that results of tests and other investigations, X-rays, etc., which were ordered after the previous visit are available.

Receiving patients

When a visitor arrives at reception you should go through the following stages.

- Smile and greet them courteously.

- Establish their identity and the reason for their visit.

- If the visitor has arrived at the wrong clinic in a busy hospital, give them clear and accurate directions and, wherever possible, provide them with an escort. This is particularly important if they are confused or distressed.

- If the visitor is a patient booked into the clinic, ask them to take a seat and explain to them:

    – which doctor will see them
    – how long they are likely to have to wait
    – where they can obtain refreshments
    – where the toilet is situated.

- Deal patiently and cheerfully with any queries the patient may have, and if you cannot answer their questions yourself, find someone (e.g. a nurse) who can.

- If there is likely to be any delay in the patient being seen, try to find out how long this is expected to be, and give the patient a diplomatic and apologetic explanation.

- If the patient has language difficulties, obtain an interpreter or linkworker.

You should always be aware that the visitor may be experiencing discomfort or may be worried about the visit. This should be taken into account in all dealings with patients, their relatives and friends.

Admissions from the waiting-list

Admissions from the waiting-list (elective admissions) are usually handled by an admissions office, which is also responsible for keeping an accurate bed state for the entire hospital. Beds are not occupied at all times, although the hospital will try to maintain occupancy to the maximum in order to make best use of resources. Elective admissions will fill a proportion of beds, but there must be the space and flexibility to be able to accommodate unforeseen demands. A pattern will have emerged over time, and the hospital will plan the use of its beds accordingly.

Admissions on to wards for day-case treatment, day surgery, or for the delivery of babies may be booked directly by those departments. Lists of expected admissions are given to each ward daily and copied to the records department so that case notes are made available.

Accident and Emergency admissions

When a patient is brought into A&E by ambulance, the drivers will pass on whatever information they have obtained, and the receptionist will check what previous records exist for that patient. Treatment will not be delayed for this information if it is urgently needed. Specific procedures are followed if the patient is a road traffic accident victim, where ambulance transport costs are recovered, usually from the driver's insurance. Special arrangements also exist for suspected non-accidental injury of a child.

Every hospital has its own procedure for major accidents, and will rehearse it in conjunction with the emergency services from time to time.

Follow-up after admission

When a patient is discharged from hospital, the medical staff prepare a form for the patient to hand to their GP. A form is also completed for financial purposes, showing the diagnosis and any operations performed. After discharge, a full summary is sent to the GP.

Not all patients leave the hospital alive. Following the death of a patient, the relatives must of course be dealt with in a kind and sensitive manner.

Home from hospital support

An increasing number of hospitals are finding that a patient can be discharged more successfully if they are offered support at home for a period of time following their return. Home from hospital teams consist of trained nurses and care support staff who arrange to visit frequently and regularly over a specified period to help the patient to adjust to being back at home. Help is offered with a range of activities designed to increase the patient's confidence in being able to cope at home. A speedier and more successful discharge both helps the patient and keeps acute hospital beds available for those who need acute nursing care.

Day cases and ward attendees

More and more people opt for surgery as a day case where this is possible. Strict criteria apply, and not all procedures or all patients can be dealt with in this way. Every effort is made to ensure that the patient has someone to collect them at the end of the day. An overnight stay will always be available should the patient's condition require it.

Most hospitals have taken steps to increase the proportion of work done on a day-case basis but, interestingly, the assumption frequently made by patients that this is a cheaper option for the NHS is not often borne out. Many hospitals find that variable costs for tests, disposables, etc., are higher per patient, and since they will be putting more patients through each bed (one per day rather than, for example, one per two or three days), total costs for these items can escalate. Staff costs can be higher because of the greater dependency of each patient, and the fixed costs associated with the building are not reduced until there has been a major shift from inpatients to day cases, allowing ward closures and large staff reductions.

The hospital team

Hospital staff fall into a number of professional groups, as described below.

Medical staff

- *Consultants* are responsible for the diagnosis and treatment of patients referred to them.

- *Junior doctors in training*, house-officers, senior house-officers and specialist registrars, work for a consultant's firm. Although they are qualified doctors, they are in training for specialist roles.

- *Other doctors*, such as staff grades, clinical assistants, hospital practitioners and associate specialists, are also attached to a consultant's firm. They are below consultant grade but are no longer in training.

Nursing staff

- *Nurses and midwives* provide the regular care for patients as set out in the care plan, and administer drugs and treatment under the direction of the doctor. Psychiatric nurses work to ensure patients' mental health. Midwives care for mothers and babies and have special status as independent practitioners, which allows them in certain circumstances to practise without a doctor's prior instruction.

- *Healthcare assistants* and nursing assistants work with qualified nurses and therapists to deliver non-technical care to patients.

- *Nurse practitioners* are nurses with specific training to allow them to practise independently, in some cases taking on responsibilities that are usually held by junior doctors. They may run clinics, assess priorities in A&E departments (known as triage), and undertake some treatments.

Therapy staff

- *Physiotherapists* diagnose and treat patients' difficulties with movement and rehabilitation after illness or injury, using exercises, manipulation and a range of equipment.

- *Occupational therapists* help patients to resume a normal life through activity-based treatments and the provision of aids to living, such as special tools and appliances.

- *Dietitians* advise patients and other care staff on the best food and drink for particular conditions. They also advise on intravenous and other drip-feeding procedures.

- *Speech and language therapists* help patients with communication difficulties, especially after a stroke or other injury to the head, throat or chest. They also treat children who have communication difficulties.

- *Hearing therapists* assist patients with hearing difficulties and support those with hearing aids.

- *Pharmacists* provide specialist advice on appropriate drug treatments, including drug interactions, and supply drugs to inpatients and outpatients.

Diagnostic staff

- *Pathology staff* carry out a range of tests which are grouped into categories. Haematology staff perform tests on blood. Cytology staff study the nature of cells (especially cancerous or other diseased ones). Histology staff study tissues to detect disease. Microbiology staff test urine, faeces and other body fluids for parasites and bacteria. Virology staff look for the presence of viruses. Chemistry staff look for the presence of chemicals which may cause illness or be a symptom of disease.

- *Radiography staff* take X-rays for interpretation by a radiologist. They perform various treatments, such as barium meals or dye injections, to show up particular parts of the body. They also use ultrasound to examine babies in the womb, and to detect disease (e.g. a tumour) in other parts of the body. Computer axial tomography (CAT) scanning uses a computer to reconstruct an image of a layer of tissue in the body. Nuclear magnetic resonance imaging (NMRI) uses radio frequency radiation and a magnetic field to produce anatomical sections of the body.

- *ECG staff* use an electrocardiograph to take readings which describe the functioning of a patient's heart, for cardiologists to interpret.

- *EEG staff* use an electroencephalograph to produce a picture of brain activity, by placing small electrodes on the patient's head to measure electrical impulses. Consultants in EEG interpret the pictures.

Support workers

- *Non-clinical support departments* include chaplaincy, catering, cleaning, porters, security, building, engineering, linen and laundry, and transport.

Management and administration

- *Management departments* include the chief executive's team, general managers, directors of nursing and midwifery, business managers, human resources, finance, payroll, information and marketing.

- *Administrative support* is provided by admissions, registry and medical records.

Clinical audit

The term 'clinical audit' embraces the audit activity of all healthcare professionals, including nurses, doctors and other healthcare staff. It is a widely used tool within hospitals, and is defined as the systematic and critical analysis of the quality of clinical care, including the procedures used for diagnosis, treatment and care, the associated resources and the resulting outcome and quality of life for the patient.

As a general principle, audit should be professionally led and should focus on improving outcomes. It will have the greatest impact if it forms part of routine clinical care. It should be seen as an educational process and be an important part of quality programmes. It must respect confidentiality at the individual patient or clinician level, and take into consideration the views of the patient and their carers.

What is a medical record?

A medical record is the history of a patient's treatment as an outpatient or inpatient, or both, at a particular hospital. If it is known that a patient has attended another hospital, a copy of that treatment record should be included in the current hospital medical record. A complete record prevents duplication and facilitates future care. In most cases, at present, the most complete medical records are the GP's notes, as they follow patients when they move around geographically. GP records should also contain details of any hospital treatment received by the patient, as well as any letters and summaries from hospitals which the patient may have attended.

Why have medical records in hospitals?

- They are of most value in the treatment of patients, as a reminder and as a means of communication to doctors, nurses, etc. of what has been given and with what effect, and investigations which have been made and the results.

- They are an educational instrument and, as such, are used to teach medical students, nurses and other students.

- They are used for research.

Storage of medical records

Every hospital has its own system, but there are three main methods:

- lateral filing systems – files are arranged side by side on shelves
- vertical filing systems – files are stored in multi-drawer cabinets
- rotary (carousel) systems.

Each of these methods has its advantages and disadvantages. The security of any area in which medical records are held is of prime importance.

Case notes

Although medical records were standardised when the NHS was instituted in order to ensure uniformity of record-keeping procedures, these vary from one hospital to another. A hospital receptionist or medical secretary who moves from one hospital to another is unlikely to find herself handling exactly the same procedures. Standardisation overall does exist but without rigidity.

Case notes basically follow the same pattern everywhere, being contained in A4-sized folders and consisting of five sections:

- identification
- medical
- nursing
- correspondence
- results (e.g. pathology tests, X-rays).

Identification section

This section allows space for the following information:

- hospital's name and code number, which is usually printed
- patient's name, address, status and telephone number
- patient's postcode
- patient's date of birth
- GP information
- consultant
- hospital number
- patient's occupation
- patient's religion
- NHS number
- next-of-kin information.

Medical section

This section is for doctors' use only, and generally consists of the following:

- history of present complaint
- past medical history (PMH)
- family history
- patient complains of (PCO)
- on examination (OE)
- differential diagnosis

- investigations
- treatment.

Nursing section

This section contains the observations of nursing staff (recorded only when patients are admitted):

- nursing record
- temperature, pulse, respiration (TPR) – graphic records on special sheets; also used for blood pressure, micturition and bowel function
- intake and output charts (record of all fluids taken orally or by transfusion and excreted).

Correspondence section

This section will usually include the following:

- GP's referral letter or pro forma referral
- consultant's reports to GP
- letters to and from other consultants or professionals.

Other information

The records may also contain the following:

- prescription charge
- social history
- theatre/surgical operation sheet
- consent form
- anaesthetic form.

The order of all these sheets inside the folder will vary from one hospital to another, and ideally the order is printed either on the front or inside the cover. Each section of the case notes is generally filed in chronological order.

Master index

In theory, each patient should have only one medical record. This rule is broken by the law which states that the records of patients who attend the genitourinary clinics must be kept separate from any other medical records belonging to such patients. Psychiatric medical records of patients are also usually kept separately, with just a note placed in the main medical record stating where and when the patient attended for psychiatric care. In order to reduce the number of patients with several medical records, a master index is kept.

The master index is an alphabetical list of patients who have attended the hospital. It can be kept on cards and filed manually, on microfiche, on computer, on microfilm or on optical disc. The information recorded is usually basic, consisting of surname, forename(s), sex, date of birth, home address, marital status, sometimes the date of first attendance and consultants seen, religion, date of death and patient index number.

The master index record for the A & E and emergency eye departments usually consists of alphabetically filed cards of attendees there.

Filing room/medical records library

This is the hub of the medical records department. It is often located on a lower-ground or ground floor because of the weight of all the records. Security in this area is of prime importance. Unauthorised access cannot be allowed.

Within the library, files will be organised according to a strict system. A number of different filing systems exist as follows, although in most hospitals medical records are filed by patient master index number. Colour coding is often used to prevent misfiling.

Master index number – terminal digit (12 34 **56**)

Six numbers are required. 12 34 **56** gives 56 as the terminal digit, 34 as the middle digit and 12 as the first digit. Divide the main area into 100 sections, 00 to 99, and these divisions give the foundation for terminal digit filing. This means that 56 will be in main section 56. The main sections are again divided into another 00 to 99 subsections, so 56 will be placed in subsection 34 and 12 will be placed behind 11 and before 13 in subsection 34. Although this may sound complicated, with a little practice it is easy to work and helps to reduce misfiling.

Middle digit (12 **34** 56)

A similar process to terminal digit is followed, but the numbers are followed in a different order:

*   straight numerical (1, 2, 3, etc.)

*   date of birth – alphabetical

*   surname – alphabetical.

Medical records procedures for departments

Accident and Emergency records

If a patient arrives in hospital by emergency ambulance, the drivers will fill in the ambulance book stating what information they have collected about the patient. A receptionist will check if there are previous A & E records and/or medical records, and will obtain them as quickly as possible. Treatment does not wait until these are found. If there is no record of previous attendance, an A&E record is started with what information is available. This may be difficult if the patient is unconscious and un-accompanied, so there must be a follow-up should the patient eventually go on to a ward. Nurses usually record any property that the patient is carrying, but a receptionist could be asked to do so, with a witness.

   If the medical record shows that the patient has current appointments for outpatients, or has been booked for admission or for theatre, these departments must be informed if the patient is not going to attend.

Outpatient records

Outpatients attend the hospital after a letter of referral from their GP. Many GPs use a referral form. This gives basic details of the patient which help to find any existing medical records. The letters go to the consultant or senior registrar of the department concerned, and an appointment is scheduled according to urgency. A list for each clinic is drawn up, and the medical records for all patients booked are then prepared.

A copy of the manual list or the computer list in 'pulling' order is produced ('pulling' is jargon for the actual gathering together of medical records from the filing shelves). Filing-room staff, clinic clerks, receptionists or admission-office staff may do this, and again this will vary according to each hospital's system.

The person preparing for the clinic will receive a copy of the list, and must obtain the medical records and laboratory tests, X-rays, etc. which were ordered at the previous visit. These results must be in the medical records and the X-rays ordered so that they are at the clinic. The medical records are also checked to ensure that there is paper on which the medical staff may write, and are 'stamped' or written up with the date and the consultant of the clinic.

If the patient is new to the hospital, the case notes are partially written up (in order to save paper and time), but the details are not confirmed on the computer until the patient has actually arrived. On arrival, all of the patient details are checked and any missing information is obtained. If a manual system is used, this information is put on the master index card.

Day-case records

These are usually handled by the department or the ward concerned. The medical records department is contacted for the necessary records before the patient arrives, where possible. The procedure is broadly the same as that described above for outpatients.

Maternity records

In many hospitals these records are retained by the woman throughout her pregnancy and only kept by the hospital after her confinement.

Admissions and transfers

Lists of expected admissions are sent to each ward daily. A copy of this list is sent to the records library so that the medical records can be on the wards before the patient is admitted. Usually the ward receptionist does the check on the contents of the medical records, as described above for outpatients.

Retention of records

The usual retention periods are as follows:

- obstetric records – 25 years, or eight years after the death of the child but not of the mother

- children and young people – until the patient's twenty-fifth birthday, or twenty-sixth if the entry was made when the young person was 17 years of age, or eight years after death if sooner (10 years for GP records)

- psychiatric patients (within meaning of Mental Health Act 1983) – 20 years after treatment is no longer considered necessary, or eight years after death (10 years for GP records)

- all other personal health records – eight years after the end of treatment (10 years for GP records).

Destruction of medical records

Medical records departments will have a written destruction policy which will have been agreed by both clinical and administrative staff.

Destruction of medical records should only be carried out by authorised personnel in accordance with the written policy, by incineration or shredding. Destruction should be monitored to ensure absolute confidentiality. A record of instruction should be retained.

What's new in medical records?

There is a trend towards permitting patients to carry their own notes. This is particularly useful in cases where patients have a chronic condition such as diabetes, or high blood pressure.

For many years, maternity patients have carried a 'co-operation' card which has proved highly successful and parent-held records are more common where young children are concerned.

It has been found that patients do not lose their records, and that being responsible for their own record may even be beneficial. The main disadvantage is that hospital records may not be complete, which could prove difficult in cases of litigation.

'Smart' cards the size of credit cards have existed for a number of years, and trials have been conducted in parts of the UK on their use to carry health records. They have also been used by pharmacies to track prescriptions. However, smart-card systems have not yet been implemented comprehensively in the NHS.

Smart cards contain a large amount of information in a small microchip, but they require sufficient locations with input devices and readers before they can be universally adopted. They are commonly used in France and other European countries for health purposes.

The computer-based electronic record has also been on trial in the UK, but it does not seem likely that electronic records will replace paper records in the foreseeable future.

The role of the secretary in hospital

The vital link

The secretary's role is a vital one in the smooth running of the department. Frequently the first point of contact, the secretary acts as a representative of those for whom she works, and also represents the whole organisation. She provides a link between members of the healthcare team, and between them and the outside world, and her involvement can ensure that scarce resources, such as a consultant's time or a theatre list, are used as efficiently as possible, and to the very best advantage. Diplomat, oiler of wheels, the one who gets things done, the one who remembers that important detail that everyone else has forgotten – the role is as varied as it is complex.

Core knowledge and skills

All secretarial posts in healthcare services require a body of core knowledge and skills which underpin all activities within the job. These include good interpersonal skills, respect for confidentiality, the ability to use appropriate medical terms, an understanding of the principles of medical ethics and etiquette, and sensitivity to the physical and psychological needs of patients and their carers.

In addition to these, there is a requirement to comply with legal requirements concerning working practices, and to be aware of and work within other health and safety regulations.

Key result areas

The role of each individual will vary, and the emphasis given to different parts of each job will be different, but the following key result areas are common to most.

- *Communications –*

  processing, distribution and despatch of mail; efficient and courteous use of communications systems, including telephone, answering machines, pagers, fax, telex and electronic mail

- *Correspondence –*

  identifying, prioritising and responding to correspondence for own action, including letters, circulars, invoices and statements; passing on correspondence for others' attention promptly

- *Organising work schedules –*

  maintaining diaries, visual planners, computerised and other scheduling aids; making and confirming appointments; planning and prioritising own work schedule; co-ordinating assistance where necessary

- *Information –*

  using manual and computerised filing systems; responding to requests for and producing information from internal and external sources, including public documents, timetables and statistics; presenting information in different formats

- *Office administration –*

  managing and controlling office stock, following appropriate ordering procedures; dealing with faulty equipment; maintaining a petty cash system

- *Meetings –*

  preparing and producing agenda papers and minutes; booking rooms, refreshments and audio-visual aids; arranging room layout; attending meetings to take notes, and producing formal records of business undertaken

- *Reception –*

  receiving and screening visitors, and assisting them wherever possible

- *Documents and reports –*

  preparing and producing documents, including reports, tables and statistics; arranging copying, collating and binding

- *Appointment systems –*   answering requests for and allocating appointments; following booking-in procedures, registration procedures, preparing case notes, paperwork, tests, results, etc. for clinics or surgical lists

- *Waiting-lists –*   accurately compiling and prioritising waiting-lists (manual or computerised); arranging and confirming appointments, handling queries and undertaking follow-up action as necessary

- *Health and safety –*   ensuring that the work area is kept free from hazards; recording and reporting accidents and unsafe features; following safe methods for lifting and handling heavy or bulky items; following procedures for raising the alarm or summoning assistance; adhering to procedures for handling specimens

- *Patient care and support –*   dealing with patients and carers with sensitivity, identifying and responding to their needs; adhering to the requirements of the Patient's Charter; arranging transport and escorts, following procedures for handling patients' property

8

Private medicine

Introduction

Throughout the development of the National Health Service, the private care sector continued to operate and remained a minor element of the total health provision, until the 1980s when it rapidly expanded in response to the various constraints on the NHS. The number of both health insurance schemes and private providers has expanded, and by 1989, 13% of the population in the UK was covered by private medical insurance, and approximately 17% of all inpatients were treated privately and 17% of elective surgery was carried out in the private sector. At the same time there has been an increase in the number of private residential and nursing homes.

A number of medical secretaries and receptionists are now employed in private medicine, either working for specialist physicians or surgeons in their consulting rooms, or in a private clinic or hospital.

Although their function is essentially similar to that of secretaries and receptionists working in NHS organisations, there are certain differences in working practice (*see* Chapters 6 and 7).

Changes in the relationship between the NHS and the private sector

The NHS Plan states that 'for years there has been a stand-off between the NHS and private sector providers of healthcare. This has to end'. As a result, the new arrangement is set out as a concordat between the NHS and the private sector, covering private and voluntary providers of healthcare. A national framework for partnership will include a set of guidelines to help primary care groups and trusts when they commission services. A patient would remain an NHS patient even if they were treated in the private sector, and as an NHS patient care would remain free at the point of delivery.

Private clinic or hospital

Patient contact and communication

Receptionists welcome patients on arrival at the clinic or hospital, where they may be asked to complete registration forms. They will then direct them to the appropriate departments, which include the following:

- outpatients
- physiotherapy
- X-ray/imaging
- pathology.

They may take telephone calls from patients, give advice on payment protocol, make an appointment for them to see a consultant or other healthcare professional and, if necessary, refer to a nurse for advice.

Facilities

Private hospitals and clinics provide patients with rooms equipped to the highest standards to ensure a relaxed and comfortable environment, which is conducive to rapid recovery and convalescence. Rooms are generally equipped with *en suite* bathroom facilities, as well as telephone and colour television. Other amenities available will probably include the following:

- library
- mail, fax and secretarial services
- counsellor (for patients and their families)
- hairdressing and laundry services
- chiropody
- private ambulances

- television, videos and personal telephones

- *en suite* bathroom facilities.

Private hospitals offer a wide range of menus, designed with 'healthy eating' in mind, and providing a nutritionally balanced diet. Light refreshments are usually available for visitors.

Operating theatres and diagnostic and treatment departments are usually equipped to the highest standards and use the latest technology. Resident medical officers provide 24-hour medical cover for patients.

Customer care

Customer care is always an important element in a private clinic. For example, tea or coffee is offered free of charge to patients who are waiting in outpatients.

In an effort to improve the quality of care, receptionists will present questionnaires to patients, who are asked to comment on all aspects of their care through the outpatient department, including reception, nursing, X-ray, phlebotomy, etc.

Other aspects of customer care are the same as would be expected from a similar NHS organisation (e.g. arranging for a wheelchair or porter, and generally helping a patient as is felt necessary).

Changes and developments

The independent acute healthcare sector has seen many changes in recent months. The increasing demands of clinical governance (*see* Chapter 13), the regulation of independent hospitals, the National Frameworks, public expectations and media interest in healthcare have all combined to provide a challenge to management teams in the private sector.

Quality assurance

Private medicine is a highly competitive market, and hospitals and clinics have accordingly developed quality assurance programmes to maintain and improve standards. Regular audits and reviews are held to monitor achievements against written standards. Patients' opinions and views are an integral part of performance audit. Staff training and development are generally included as initiatives contributing to providing expert care and attention to patients at all times.

Telephone skills

In common with other areas of medical practice, the receptionist in a private clinic or hospital deals with all types of people – elderly, vague people, overseas visitors who cannot speak English very well, impatient people and demanding people. Patience, tact, understanding and a good telephone manner are just as essential in a private setting, as well as the ability to deal with situations efficiently and quickly because there is always another call waiting to be dealt with!

Appointments

When patients make appointments, they are asked for the following basic information:

- name – surname and forename(s)
- age, if necessary
- telephone number
- address
- whether they have medical insurance.

An appointment card is sent to the patient with directions on how to reach the clinic, and details of car parking availability. The patient is informed of consultation costs (if known) and the cost of any investigations. Any special instructions that may be necessary will also be sent to patients prior to their appointments.

Outpatient hospital/clinic registration procedure

On arrival at reception, patients are asked to complete a registration form giving the following information:

- name, address and telephone number
- name of consultant
- method of payment; they may be asked to sign to confirm that they are willing to pay for their treatment on the day.

Inpatient registration

If a patient has to be admitted, a more detailed form is given to them for completion, which also asks for details of their insurance cover.

In some private clinics, patients may be encouraged to pay for outpatient treatment on the day of their appointment, and to get any insurance forms signed there and then by the consultant, so that there will be little or no delay in reimbursement.

Pathology and X-ray

Receptionists may generate accounts for patients attending for pathology and X-ray, and will request payment at the time of investigation.

Medical records

Consultants in a private hospital or clinic will bring patients' notes with them and keep them in their personal possession.

The only records that are kept at the clinic will be screening records such as well-woman, executive screening, breast screening, etc. All records of work generated by the staff are retained at the clinic.

Mail – incoming and outgoing

Mail addressed to doctors is generally kept in pigeon-holes for their collection. All outgoing mail, accounts, letters, etc., are collected by the mail room at the end of the day for posting.

Patient accounts

The preparation and processing of patient accounts is a major part of the receptionist's job. They are prepared on the computer, and have to be ready for patients when they leave the clinic. Private hospitals and clinics have the facility to collect cash, accept payment by means of credit cards and cheques, and often have a 'Switch' machine.

Systems

All accounts for the day will be sent to a main accounts department for filing. Any outstanding bills can be demonstrated on the computer screen. There is a variety of software available, but a frequently used system is 'Compucare'.

Liaison with other healthcare professionals

Receptionists have regular contact with consultants and their secretaries, as well as with physiotherapy, X-ray and nursing staff at the clinic. They will have frequent telephone contact with almost every sector of the medical field, including laboratory staff, doctors, secretaries, NHS hospitals, clinics (private and NHS), psychologists, etc.

From time to time, they may be asked to contact a patient's private medical insurance company for information about levels of cover, etc.

Waiting-areas and consulting rooms

Consulting rooms are checked and maintained by nursing staff, except for stationery items, which are the responsibility of the receptionists.

Doctors will usually liaise by telephone to ask for their patients to be taken to them, and the receptionist or nurse will show them into the doctors' rooms.

Waiting-areas are kept clean and tidy by frequent visits from housekeepers. Catering staff will ensure that there is a supply of tea and coffee and remove dirty cups from the waiting-area. Magazines are always available for patients.

The secretary in private practice

The role of the secretary in private practice is a diverse and varied one that requires qualities and skills in addition to those needed for secretarial duties. In many instances the secretary will be working on her own, apart from the days when her consultant is seeing patients at the practice. This means that decisions of a non-medical nature may have to be made.

Reception and secretarial duties

A great deal of the secretary's time is involved with answering the telephone, dealing with patients' enquiries and making appointments.

Once an appointment has been made for a new patient, a file is made up containing basic patient information and details of private medical insurance cover, in readiness for the initial consultation.

The secretary may be asked by her consultant to organise investigations (pathology, radiological examination, etc.) for patients when necessary, and to arrange for external referrals (e.g. physiotherapy, other consultants). Admission to the hospital or clinic may also be arranged for the patient.

From time to time the secretary will need to liaise with her NHS counterpart, either to leave a message or to contact the consultant when he or she is working in the hospital department.

She will be responsible for keeping the consulting-room, waiting-room and her own office tidy and generally ensuring the comfort of patients while they are waiting to see the doctor.

It is advisable for the secretary to ensure that patients are made aware of the costs involved in private treatment for both self-paying individuals and those with health insurance. Patients who will be undergoing surgery must be informed of the procedure codes and the expected fees for the surgeon, anaesthetist and any others involved. It should also be mentioned that if any additional procedure is performed, it will be reflected in their final account. Insured patients must be advised to contact their company in order to obtain authorisation for the procedure, and to find out whether there is likely to be a shortfall on the fees. This is not within the remit of the secretary, as the policy is between the insurance company and the patient, *not* between the company and the consultant, but the secretary may need to contact the company in a supporting role.

Some insurance companies are now offering direct invoicing and payment through electronic data interchange (EDI). The latter is an established method for sending messages directly from one computer system to another, particularly business transactions. Some insurance companies have set up their own electronic billing systems.

Clerical duties

On a daily basis mail has to be sorted and incoming correspondence attended to as appropriate. Photocopying of insurance or medical reports may be necessary from time to time, and messages sent or received by facsimile (fax) transmission dealt with accordingly. Correspondence will have to be posted and a supply of postage stamps maintained at the practice.

The secretary will usually be responsible for petty cash for purchasing office sundries and maintaining supplies of stationery and other items.

She will pull patients' records prior to consultation and check that the results of investigations previously requested are complete. Following consultation and any further action that has to be taken, the notes will be filed away.

Email messages (both incoming and outgoing) are becoming a popular means of communication. The receptionist or secretary should always check for messages at least twice a day.

On a daily basis, too, all incoming cheques and cash should be checked against the outstanding patient accounts.

Secretarial skills

Good secretarial skills are important, including typing and competent use of word-processing systems. Many consultants prefer to dictate their letters and reports on to a dictating machine, but some still prefer their secretaries to use shorthand. Usually a combination of shorthand and audiotyping skills is desirable.

A knowledge of medical terminology and medical abbreviations is always useful, but not necessarily essential. A good medical dictionary, common sense and an ability to learn the specialist terms will usually suffice.

In private practice, with no nurse in attendance, the secretary may be asked to act as a chaperone during the consultant's examination of the patient.

Practice management

The secretary in private practice will find that, in addition to her other duties, she is also a practice manager. The good manager will update existing systems to ensure that the practice operates effectively and in an efficient way. She will be responsible for sending patient accounts and, if necessary, will remind patients that settlement of their outstanding account is overdue, and will follow up unpaid accounts on a regular basis, as well as patient account reconciliation. Any long-standing overdue accounts will be referred to a debt collection agency when necessary.

At least once a week, all cheques and cash should be entered in the accounts book and paid into the bank. An accounts book should also be kept for recording income and outgoings for office supplies, catering, etc.

The secretary will reconcile the petty cash account on a regular (usually monthly) basis, and will recommend when accounts should be paid by the consultant.

Another financial aspect of the work of the medical secretary in private practice will no doubt be to operate a payroll (perhaps for only one person), to calculate her own PAYE and NI contributions, and to make year end returns to the Inland Revenue. She will also be responsible for ordering any supplies necessary for the doctor's consulting room and her own office requirements.

Summary

It will be noted that the role of the receptionist and secretary in private practice is very similar to that of their counterpart working in an NHS organisation, but with greater financial and accounting responsibilities.

An essential quality is to be able to deal with patients in an efficient yet sympathetic manner, and to understand the emotions and concerns experienced by patients when they enter a clinical environment. Although it is desirable for secretaries and receptionists to have a knowledge of medical terminology and other clinical aspects, a competent person will learn these as they carry out their day-to-day duties.

9

Forms, fees and finances in general practice

Introduction

General medical practice is a small business, like any other practice of professionals (e.g. solicitors or accountants). Therefore there is a need to get money in to cover the costs of providing the service to patients. Figure 9.1 shows a list of expenses incurred in running a practice and a list of sources of income. The profit is the difference between income and expenditure, and it is from the profit that the partners take their drawings. It is therefore easy to understand why doctors insist that all claims for payments are made promptly and that expenses are kept to a minimum.

The majority of the income is via the health authority/health board/ health and social services board, and in order to claim its share, a practice has to complete a variety of forms – these are the equivalent of invoices for services given. Although some of the forms are filled in only when a partner joins a practice, or on an annual basis, the majority are completed as each service is rendered. Therefore the receptionist is a key person in ensuring that forms are completed as patients enter or leave the premises. Figure 9.2 shows the items of income set against the staff members who may be responsible for ensuring that the claim forms are completed.

Practices have a variety of ways of sharing out the clerical workload, and in larger practices it may be expedient to have one or two staff who take responsibility for checking that forms are completed and sent off to the health authority/health board/health and social services board on a regular basis. However, if all of the receptionists are competent at completing the forms accurately and completely, the task of batching and sending off becomes much easier and quicker.

Income

NHS   **Basic practice allowance (BPA)**
(a sliding scale, based on number of patients)
Additions made to BPA:

Practice in designated area (Types 1 and 2)
Seniority allowance (based on number of years)
Qualified and years working as a GP
(e.g. 5, 10, 19, 25 years)
Initial practice allowance
Associate allowance
Deprivation payments (for GPs providing
services to a deprived area); the new
system enumerates payments into four
Bands (Band 4, 3, 2, 1)
Associate allowance (based on number of
years)

Capitation fees
• Under 65 years
• 65–74 years
• 75 years and over

Health promotion activities
Dispensing payments
Postgraduate education allowance
Medical students

Chronic disease management programme
(a) Diabetic allowance
(b) Asthma allowance

PRIVATE
Private medical attendant form
Insurance medicals
Cremation forms
Private medical certificates

OTHER APPOINTMENTS
Company or school medical officer
Police surgeon

Items of service
Registration
Child health surveillance
Night payments
(annual fee/consultation fee)
Maternity services
Emergency treatment
Immediately necessary treatment
Minor surgery
Temporary residents
Adult vaccination/immunisation

Target payments
Cervical cytology*
Immunisations under twos*
Immunisations under fives*

*Payable at lower and higher rates

Reimbursements
Registrar's salary
GP registrar's scheme
Rent and rates
Staff salaries and National Insurance
Computer maintenance
Staff training

SUNDRY
Passport forms
Travel vaccinations (e.g. yellow fever)
PSV, HGV, elderly driver
Private pilot's licence

	Expenditure
Practice	Drugs and instruments
	Hire and maintenance of equipment
	Repairs and renewals
Premises	Rates and water rates
	Heat and light
	Insurance
	Cleaning
Salaries	Staff
	Registrar
Administration	Postage
	Stationery
	Telephone
Professional fees	Accountant
	Solicitor
Banking	Interest
	Loan repayments

The turnover (i.e. all forms of income added together) of a large practice may be in excess of £600 000 whereas that of a small single-handed practice might be £100 000.

Figure 9.1   Practice income and expenditure.

Source of income	Item	Persons likely to complete the claim form			
		Receptionist	Clerk	Secretary	Manager
NHS	Practice allowance	Automatic (only affected by change of partnership)			
	Capitation				
	Registration	✔	✔		✔
	Child health surveillance	✔	✔		✔
	Deprivation	Automatic (depends upon banding)			
	Items of service				
	Registration medical	✔			
	Night visit payments	✔	✔		
	Maternity services	✔			
	Emergency treatment	✔			
	Immediately necessary treatment	✔			
	Contraceptive services	✔			
	Temporary residents	✔			
	Adult vaccination/ immunisation	✔			
	Minor surgery	✔	✔		✔
	Targets				
	Cervical cytology	✔	✔		✔
	Immunisations, under twos	✔	✔		✔
	Immunisations, under fives	✔	✔		✔
	Health-promotion banding		✔		✔
	Dispensing payments		✔		✔
	Associate allowance			✔	✔
	Seniority	Automatic once set up			✔
	Postgraduate education allowance			✔	✔
	Registrar supervision grant			✔	✔
	Medical students			✔	✔
	Reimbursements				
	Trainee salary				✔
	Rent and rates			✔	✔
	Staff salaries and National Insurance				✔
	Staff training				✔
	Computer maintenance				✔
Private	Private medical attendant reports			✔	✔
	Insurance medicals			✔	
	Cremation forms			✔	
	Sundry				
	Passport forms	✔			
	Travel vaccinations, (e.g. yellow fever)	✔			
	PSV, HVG, elderly driver	✔			
	Other appointments				
	Company or school medical officer			✔	
	Police surgeon			✔	

Figure 9.2   Income in general practice and the role of the receptionist.

General practitioners are independent contractors, and as such are self-employed and have autonomy to run their practices as they wish within the requirements of their Terms of Service.

Their income is derived from a system of fees and allowances, and those currently paid to general practitioners are set out in the Statement of Fees and Allowances (SFAs), referred to as *The Red Book* (*see* Figure 9.1 and 9.2). Figure 9.1 summarises the most relevant fees and allowances payable to GPs.

Most practices have systems for ensuring that forms are filled in at the right time. These will range from stickers on the outside of the medical record, through cardex boxes (for manual recording) to computer-generated lists and reminder messages on the computer screen when a patient record is opened. The introduction of the health authority/GP Links project whereby claims can be sent automatically to the health authority/health board/health and social services board will eventually make the paper claims redundant.

Regardless of the system of claiming, it is important that receptionists are aware of what claims should be made under what circumstances. Various publications exist which provide information on capitation, item-of-service claims, targets and payments to doctors. The most important of these is *The Red Book* – the statement of fees and allowances.

To understand what can be claimed and under what circumstances, there is no real substitute for *The Red Book* – the Statement of Fees and Allowances. This is a loose-leaf document which is updated as rates of pay, conditions regulating payments or other changes are made, and the authorising authority bases their decision regarding payments on its content. Every partner and registrar GP in a practice is issued with their own copy of *The Red Book*, and it is helpful if a copy is available to practice staff, who can then clarify any queries with the health authority/health board/health and social services board or primary care trusts. Many authorities run short courses so that practice staff can learn what the forms are for, how they should be completed, and when to return them to the appropriate authority. Staff are always willing to help receptionists with any clarification they may need, and it is often possible to make an appointment to meet the staff who deal with claims. The receptionist who regularly contacts staff in these authorities for clarification is the one who will be able to submit claims efficiently and keep abreast of trends and changes. There are numerous changes affecting primary healthcare at the present time, and networking is therefore an important activity. It is essential that all copies of *The Red Book* are kept up to date, so that when the latest SFA (amendment to *The Red Book*) is issued the new pages are appropriately filed into place and the old versions disposed of.

In the surgery a collection of claim forms can be put into a folder together with brief details of when claims should be made, notes on completing the forms, and in-house systems for recording 'due to sign again' dates. This is a useful in-house reference source and training tool for new staff. However, as and when changes are made to claims it is important to ensure that the folder is updated.

When handling claim forms and target sheets, it is important to be systematic, and therefore it is preferable not to work on reception duties at the same time, trying to fit in the paperwork between other tasks. Paperwork requires a different set of skills to those used when receiving patients. If a receptionist works a busy morning shift on the reception desk it will be almost impossible to switch from pressured reception duties to calmly working through a pile of papers without a transitionary period – a cup of coffee, popping out to the shops for some fresh air, or a chat – to wind down from the pressure.

Box 9.1

RECEPTION DESK DUTIES

Require the ability to juggle many important priorities at once

Answering the telephone, controlling surgery flow and dealing with queries are 'demand driven' activities

CLERICAL DUTIES

Require a systematic orderly approach

Processing massive piles of paper requires self-motivation – 'self driven'

Note: It is appreciated that the duties of receptionists do vary considerably from one practice to another, and that they may not all be involved in completing, recording and despatching item-of-service claim forms. In some medical practices this function is performed by the practice manager or administrator.

Practice income

Income to the practice is derived both from NHS sources and from private sources (e.g. item-of-service claim forms come via the NHS, whereas medical attendant reports for insurance companies are a private source) (*see* Figure 9.1).

The fees payable for NHS payments are shown in *The Red Book* and the BMA recommends fees for private services. Both of these sets of fees are summarised and displayed in tabular form in the doctor's weekly or monthly magazines and journals.

It is important that all sources of income are properly documented and claimed. The role of the receptionist cannot be overestimated in ensuring that services given are recorded and claimed for. The receptionist is the person who deals with the patients, is aware of what the doctor says he or she has done for a specific patient, and is therefore the pivotal person who ensures that claims are made or invoices are raised. The receptionist may not be required to do these tasks but to ensure that someone else has the necessary information to be able to do so.

However, there will be occasions when a receptionist is asked to advise a patient about what payment is required, to receive the payment and issue a receipt. Information about current fees should be kept readily to hand, together with printed receipts that only need to have the name of the patient, service given, date, amount paid and signature filled in by hand. The payment should then be passed to the appropriate person for banking.

Although most doctors are aware that private fees are a significant supplement to their income, some are reluctant to talk to patients about the fee for their services. Staff should also be aware that sums received from patients (large or small, cheque or cash) must all be passed through the practice accounts. Private fees are not a 'perk' – the Inland Revenue have been known to trace payments back over a number of years and claim back tax on them.

As in all of the other aspects of general medical practice, the receptionist has a vital role to play in the financial success of a practice by cutting down on unnecessary wastage and expense, and ensuring that all income is claimed and processed promptly.

Helpful hints for completing health authority/health board claim forms

The following information should help you complete any claim forms for which you are responsible in your practice.

Fewer better forms

On 1 July 1996 four new forms for the registration of family doctor services and items-of-service claims replaced 19 old forms. Their introduction was a result of the NHS scrutiny of bureaucracy in primary care, described in the NHS report *Patients Not Paper*.

The report found that general medical practices were overburdened by excessive paperwork. Contained in the 65 recommendations were proposals for a radical reduction in the number of forms required by general medical practices and health authorities to process patient registration and items-of-service claims.

The new forms and procedures were extensively piloted in England and Wales. In response to comments from the pilot authorities and practices, a number of changes were incorporated into the design of the forms. Logical, user-friendly and multi-purpose, they can readily be used with a minimum of training.

The forms are purchased in bulk by health authorities and supplied free of charge to practices. They are used throughout England and Wales. (Welsh-language versions are available for GMS1 and GMS2.) There are no local variations of the form and no locally produced versions of the national form.

The forms

The four forms are as follows:

*   GMS1 – family doctor services registration
*   GMS2 – maternity medical services
*   GMS3 – temporary services
*   GMS4 – items-of-service multi-claims.

There is an optional envelope, the GMS/E, which can be used for submitting claims.

Health authority/general practitioner electronic links

Practices that are electronically linked for registration only use all of the forms, retaining GMS1 as their record of the 'contract' to supply services.

Practices that are electronically linked for items of service continue to use GMS1, GMS2 and GMS3. GMS4 is used for those services that are not yet incorporated into the electronic links.

GMS1: family doctor services registration (*see* Figure 9.3)

This is to be used:

*   for an application to join a family doctor's list by a patient, child or someone who is unable to complete the form themselves
*   for an application for a child to register for child health surveillance
*   for an application to join the NHS organ donor register.

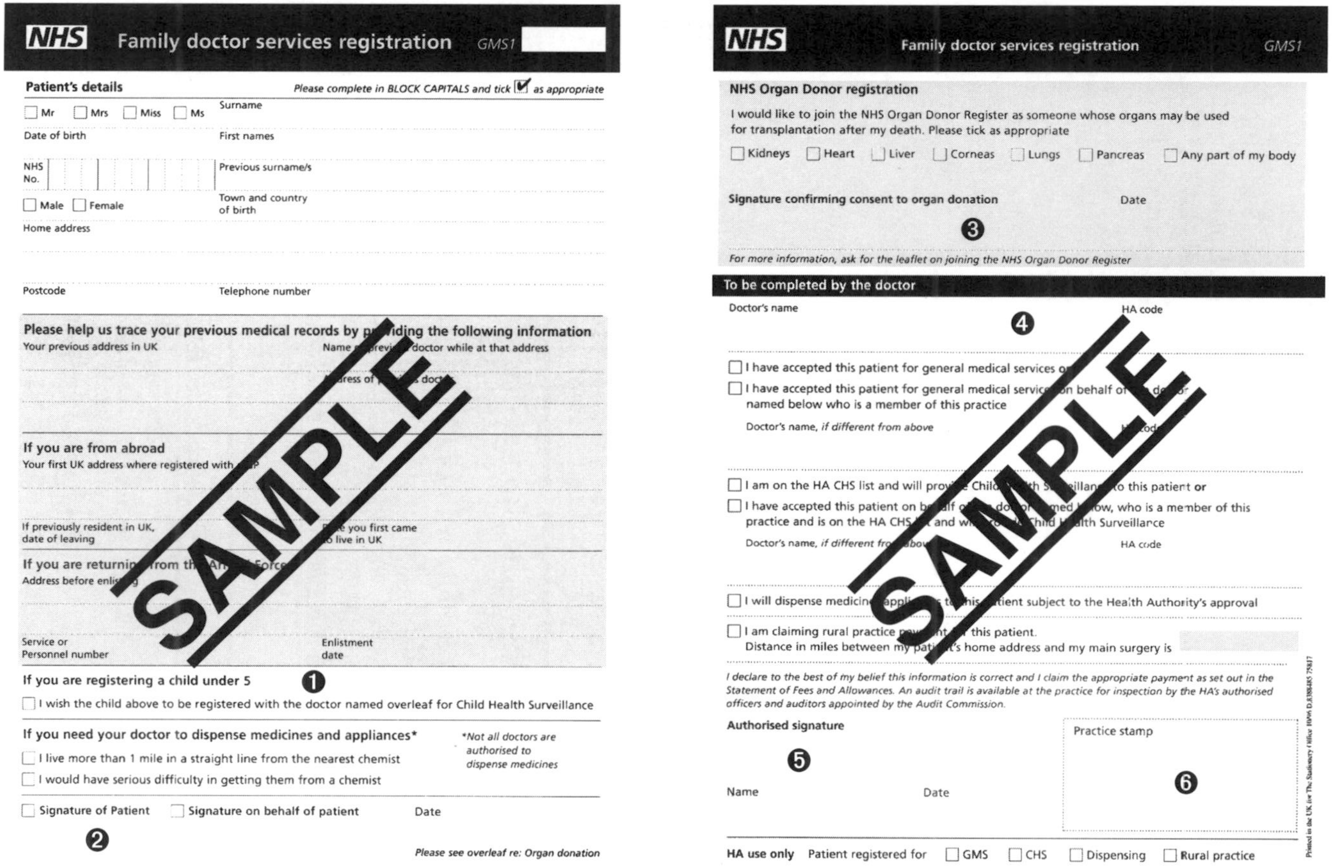

Figure 9.3   Family doctor services registration – Form GMS1.

At the practice

1   *Child health surveillance* – the form can only be used for child health surveillance claims. Under these circumstances no patient's signature is required.

2   *Patient's signature* – if the forms are completed on behalf of the patient by the doctor or practice staff, ask the patient or a patient representative to check all entries before signing GMS1. This signature should only be requested on completion of the form.

3   *NHS organ donor registration* – explain the purpose of registration, pointing out that, in the event of a patient's death, relatives' permission would be sought. If patients are undecided, give them the NHS organ donor register leaflet for further consideration. There is no upper or lower age limit, and the signature may be that of the patient or the patient's representative.

4   *HA code* – this is the GP's unique identifying code assigned to him or her by the health authority (HA).

5   *Authorised signature* – ensure that the declaration is read before signing.

6   *Practice stamp* – this is a space for the practice stamp or for entering the name of the practice.

All GMS1 forms can be submitted to the GP's responsible HA. At the HA, GMS1 forms received from practices for patients who live in neighbouring authorities are forwarded to those authorities for processing.

If electronically linked, retain the form for nine months at the practice. Otherwise send it to the HA.

GMS2: maternity medical services (*see* Figure 9.4)

Use this for the patient's application to register with the family or other GP for maternity medical services. This form replaces FP24 and FP24A.

At the practice

1   *Patient's signature* – if forms are completed on behalf of the patient by the doctor or practice staff, ask the patient or their representative to check all entries before signing GMS2. This signature should only be requested on completion of the form.

The patient's signature may be omitted if treatment is given in circumstances (e.g. a miscarriage) where the doctor considers it necessary in the patient's interest not to ask for their signature. In this

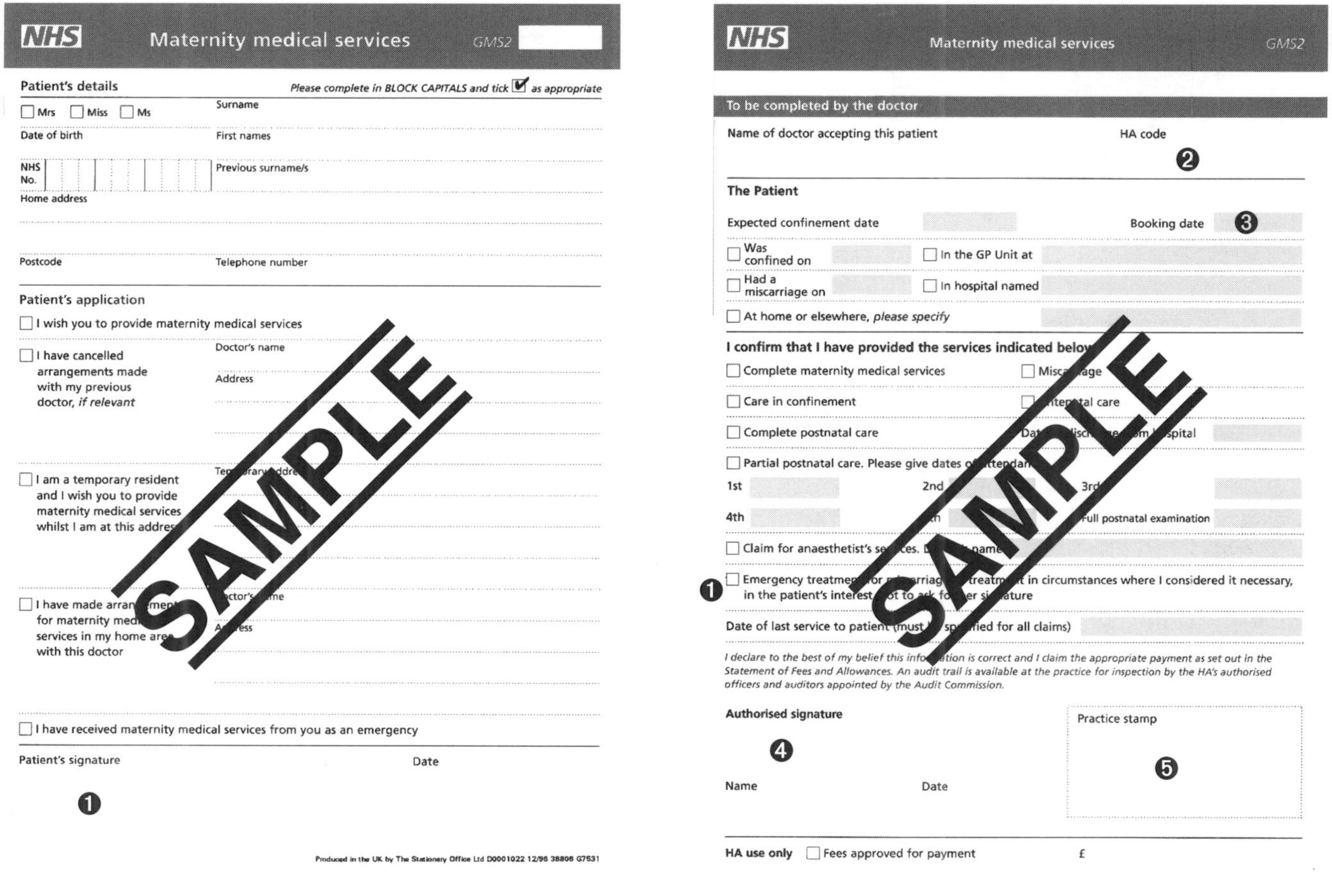

NHS Maternity medical services GMS2

Patient's details *Please complete in BLOCK CAPITALS and tick ☑ as appropriate*

☐ Mrs ☐ Miss ☐ Ms Surname

Date of birth First names

NHS No. Previous surname/s

Home address

Postcode Telephone number

Patient's application

☐ I wish you to provide maternity medical services

☐ I have cancelled arrangements made with my previous doctor, *if relevant* Doctor's name Address

☐ I am a temporary resident and I wish you to provide maternity medical services whilst I am at this addres… Te…orary addre…

☐ I have made arran…ment… for maternity med… services in my home are… with this doctor …ctor's …me A…ess

☐ I have received maternity medical services from you as an emergency

Patient's signature ❶ Date

Produced in the UK by The Stationery Office Ltd D0001022 12/96 38806 G7631

NHS Maternity medical services GMS2

To be completed by the doctor

Name of doctor accepting this patient HA code ❷

The Patient

Expected confinement date Booking date ❸

☐ Was confined on ☐ In the GP Unit at

☐ Had a miscarriage on ☐ In hospital named

☐ At home or elsewhere, *please specify*

I confirm that I have provided the services indicated belo…

☐ Complete maternity medical services ☐ Misc…age

☐ Care in confinement ☐ …te…tal care

☐ Complete postnatal care Da… …isc… …m …spital

☐ Partial postnatal care. Please give dates o… …ttendan…

1st 2nd 3rd

4th …h …ull postnatal examination

☐ Claim for anaesthetist's se…ces. … …name

❶ ☐ Emergency treatme… for … …rriag… treatm…t in circumstances where I considered it necessary, in the patient's interest, …ot to …k fo… …er si…ature

Date of last service to patient (must … sp…ified for all claims)

I declare to the best of my belief this info…ation is correct and I claim the appropriate payment as set out in the Statement of Fees and Allowances. An audit trail is available at the practice for inspection by the HA's authorised officers and auditors appointed by the Audit Commission.

Authorised signature ❹ Practice stamp ❺

Name Date

HA use only ☐ Fees approved for payment £

Figure 9.4 Maternity medical services – Form GMS2.

case, the doctor should tick the appropriate box on the reverse side of the form.

2   *HA code* – this is the GP's unique identifying code assigned to him or her by the HA.

3   *Booking date* – the booking date is the date of the doctor's acceptance.

4   *Authorised signature* – ensure that the declaration is read before signing.

5   *Practice stamp* – this is a space for the practice stamp or for entering the name of the practice.

The forms should be submitted to the GP's responsible HA. At the HA, GMS2 forms received from practices for patients who live elsewhere will be forwarded to those authorities for processing.

If electronically linked for items of service, retain the form for two years at the practice. Otherwise send to the HA.

GMS3: temporary services (*see* Figure 9.5)

Use this form for all claims for non-registered patients except those receiving minor surgery and maternity medical services. This form replaces FP19, FP106, FP32 and FP1003, and is used in place of FP81, FP82 and FP73 for non-registered patients. The form is carbonised to allow the duplication of patient details, and space is provided on the reverse side for clinical records which can be forwarded to the patient's home GP. This is a multi-claim form and can be used for more than one service per form, but only for one patient.

At the practice

1   *Doctor to whom details of treatment given should be sent* – in the case of armed services personnel, this space should be used to record the current medical centre.

2   *Authorised signature* – ensure that the declaration is read before signing.

3   *Practice stamp* – this is a space for the practice stamp or for entering the name of the practice.

4   *Clinical records* – use the space provided to record details of treatment given, including if appropriate the type of vaccination/immunisation. These details will be passed on to the patient's home doctor.

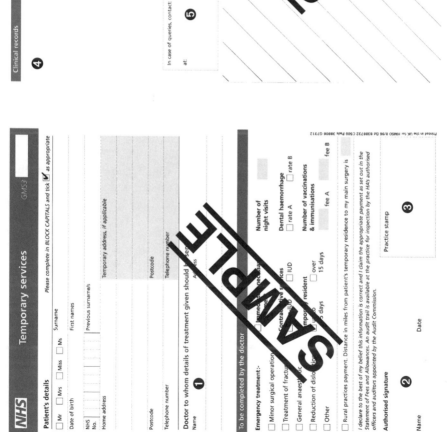

Figure 9.5   Temporary services – Form GMS3.

5 *In case of queries* – enter the name of the doctor who should be contacted in case of queries by the patient's home doctor, and enter the practice address or stamp.

6 Do not write on this area, as it will affect the legibility of the patient's details on the reverse side of the form.

Note: The patient's signature is not required on GMS3.

If electronically linked for items of service, retain the form for two years. Otherwise send it to the HA.

GMS4: items of service multi-claim (*see* Figure 9.6)

This form is used to claim for registration examination, night consultation, vaccinations and immunisations, contraceptive services, minor surgery, anaesthetic or dental haemorrhage. It replaces FP31, FP81, FP82, FP73, FP1001 and FP1002. For non-registered patients use the form GMS3, except in the case of minor surgery.

At the practice

1 *Item of service* – tick relevant box next to one item of service, then use this form *only* for the item ticked.

2 *Date* – enter the date of examination, visit, acceptance, renewal or procedure.

3 *Patient's name, date of birth and NHS number* – enter for all claims *except* minor surgery. To help speed payment, enter the patient's date of birth and NHS number.

4 The columns A and B are used to identify appropriate fee types:

- vaccinations and immunisations: enter the number of items in column A or B for the appropriate fee band

- contraceptive services: tick column A for non-IUD/tick column B for IUD/for continuous claims enter 'C' instead of a tick in column A or B

- minor surgery: claims must be grouped in fives and the patient's name and details should be omitted. Enter the procedure code in column A: I = injection; A = aspiration; N = incision; E = excision; C = cautery; O = other

- dental haemorrhage: enter a tick in column A or B for the appropriate rate band.

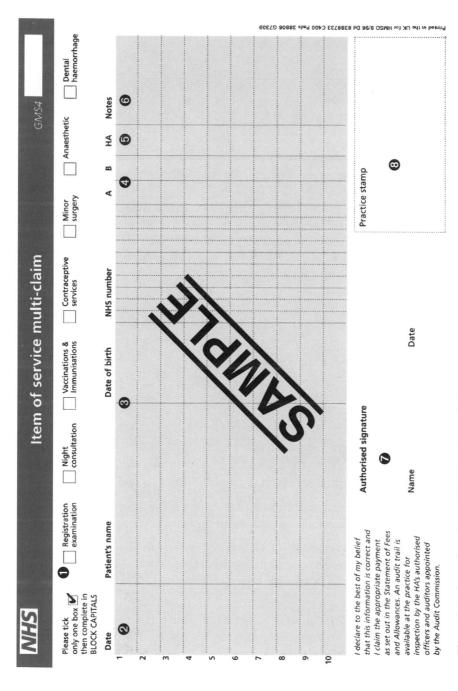

Figure 9.6 Item of service multi-claim – Form GMS4.

6 *HA column* – enter the HA in whose area the patient lives if it is outside your HA (this information is not needed for minor surgery claims).

7 *Notes* – where a continuous claim for contraceptive services is made, enter the date of the patient's previous acceptance by the doctor in this column. This column may also be used to enter other notes (e.g. to indicate that a patient should not be contacted without prior reference to their GP).

8 *Authorised signature* – please ensure that the declaration is read before signing.

9 *Practice stamp*.

GMS/E: claims summary (*see* Figure 9.7)

Use of this envelope is optional for the summarising and submission of claims to the HA.

Adult vaccination claims (FP73 (MULTI))

This form provides for up to 20 adult vaccination claims at a time. It should not be used for patients aged 16 years or under. Please ensure that the reason why vaccination is given is entered on the form (*see* Figure 9.8).

Vaccination claims (FP73)

This form should be used for vaccination claims for non-targeted children (i.e. those 5–16 years of age) (*see* Figure 9.9).

Notification of immunisations for targeted children (five years and under) (FP73/3/GP and FP73/2/GP)

Form FP73/3/GP (primary immunisations)

This form is in four parts. The top sheet records the child's personal details and the first dose of immunisation and, once completed, should be sent to the health authority. The remaining parts are retained to record the second and third doses. The second sheet retains the details from the first

NHS   **Claims summary**   *GMS/E* [   ]

Please list enclosures of claims and registrations.
All claims need NHS number and date of birth to speed payment.

Item of service multi-claims summary

		Number of claims	HA only
Registration medical examination			
Night visit			
Vaccinations & Immunisations	A		
	B		
Contraceptive services — Non-IUD	A		
IUD	B		
Minor surgery (number of sessions not procedures)			
Anaesthetic			
Dental haemorrhage			

I am also enclosing

	Number of forms	HA only
Family doctor services registration/		
Maternity medical services claim/s		
Temporary services claim/s		

SAMPLE

Date of submission

In case of query contact

Practice stamp

Printed in the UK for HMSO – Dd. 8388395, 750,000 5/96

Figure 9.7   Claims summary – Form GMS/E.

CROYD FAMILY HEALTH SERVICES AUTHORITY

FP73 (MULTI)

ADULT VACCINATION AND IMMUNISATION CLAIM (not for childhood immunisations)

Surname & Initials	Address	NHS No.	Date of Birth	Antigen	Batch No.	1, 2, 3 Reinf	Date Given	Reason (see below)	FP19 Y/N	FHSA use
1.										
2.										
3.										
4.										
5.										
6.										
7.										
8.										
9.										

SAMPLE

REASONS CODES: (a) routine measure (b) belonging to a group exposed to special risk (c) traveller abroad
(please enter name of country with code)
(d) recommended by the Community Physician/Proper Officer during an out break of disease.

PRACTICE STAMP

CLAIMING DOCTOR ....   SIGNATURE ....

Figure 9.8   Adult vaccination claims – FP73 (MULTI).

					F.P. 73 (Revised 12/88)		
VACCINATION AND IMMUNISATION ATTENDANCE AT:				CLINIC/SURGERY:			
SURNAME:				SEX: MALE/FEMALE			
FORENAMES:				D.O.B.:			
ADDRESS:				POST CODE:			
SCHOOL:		NHS NO.:		CHILD HEALTH NO.:			
GENERAL PRACTITIONER'S SURNAME AND INITIALS:							
HEALTH VISITOR'S CASE LIST NO.: ☐☐☐		(OR HV'S NAME:			)		

I consent to my child receiving the following immunisations:

Poliomyelitis	Diphtheria	Tetanus	Whooping Cough	Measles	Mumps	Rubella
☐	☐	☐	☐	☐	☐	☐

Signature of Parent of Guardian .... Date ....

TO BE COMPLETED BY PERSON ADMINISTERING IMMUNISATION:

Primary Courses		BATCH NO.	DOSE	DATE	NAME	DESIG.	STAFF ID NO.
First Dose	Diphtheria						
	Tetanus						
	Pertussis						
	Poliomyelitis						
Others (please specify)	1.						
	2.						
Second Dose	Diphtheria						
	Tetanus						
	Pertussis						
	Poliomyelitis						
Others (please specify)	1.						
	2.						
Third Dose	Diphtheria						
	Tetanus						
	Pertussis						
	Poliomyelitis						
Others (specify)	Measles						
	Mumps						
	Rubella						
Boosters	Diphtheria						
	Tetanus						
	Polio						
Others (please specify)	1.						
	2.						

Date and Result of any test of Immunity for Rubella:

Comments:

TO BE COMPLETED BY GENERAL PRACTITIONER CLAIMING PAYMENT

Name and address of General Practitioner (BLOCK CAPITALS OR STAMP)

Vaccinated as ☐ (a) A routine Measure

☐ (b) Belonging to a group exposed to special risk

(Please tick) ☐ (c) A traveller to .... (Name of Country)

☐ (d) Recommended by the Proper Officer during an outbreak of disease

I certify that the patient has been vaccinated as indicated above and I claim the appropriate fees.

Date .... Signature of Doctor ....

No: ☐☐☐☐☐

Signature of Assistant or Locum on behalf of Doctor ....

PLEASE SUBMIT THIS FORM TO THE IMMUNISATION DEPARTMENT, 12-18 LENNARD ROAD, AS SOON AS EACH DOSE IS GIVEN. PLEASE DO NOT WAIT FOR COMPLETION OF A COURSE.

NB This form has now been modified to include meningitis C.

Figure 9.9   Vaccination claims – FP73.

CROYD COMMUNITY HEALTH/GP — IMMUNISATION RECORD

Surname	Forenames		Sex	D O B		CHS No.
			M/F			

Address		Surgery/Clinic/Home/School

GP Name & Initials	HV Name	HV (CHS) No.	NHS No.

FOR PRIMARY IMMUNISATIONS ONLY

CONSENT BY PERSON WITH PARENTAL RESPONSIBILITY:

I consent to my child receiving these immunisations

Diphtheria ☐	Whooping Cough ☐	
Tetanus ☐	Hib ☐	Signed: .... Date: ....
Poliomyelitis ☐		

1ST DOSE - DELETE ANTIGEN(S) NOT GIVEN. DETAILS OF 2ND & 3RD DOSES MUST BE SHOWN ON SUBSEQUENT COPIES

	ANTIGEN	BATCH No.	DATE	NAME	STAFF ID OR DESIGNATION
1	Dip/Tet/Pert				
1	Oral Polio				
1	Hib				

FP/73/3/GP
(revised 2/92)

Figure 9.10   Notification of immunisations for targeted children – FP73/3/GP.

sheet and provides space for the second dose details. Once completed, this sheet should be sent to the health authority. The third sheet retains details from the first two sheets and provides space for the third dose to be recorded, and it should then be passed on as before. The remaining sheet (card) is the file copy and is for retention by the GP for inclusion in his or her files (*see* Figure 9.10).

Form FP73/2/GP (MMR, boosters and *ad hoc*)

This form is in two parts. Once completed, the top sheet should be passed on to the health authority. The remaining sheet is the file copy and can be used by the GP for his or her records (*see* Figure 9.11).

Post-payment verification

In place of most prepayment checking, HAs will now pay the claims submitted by practices and undertake post-payment verification of claims. This process should not be seen as mistrust of practices, but rather as an opportunity to provide practices with greater freedom whilst maintaining probity and ensuring that HAs fulfil the obligation with public money.

IMMUNISATION RECORD

Surname		Forenames		Sex	D O B		CHS No.
				M/F			

Address		Surgery/Clinic/Home

GP Name & Initials	HV Name	HV (CHS) No.	NHS No.

NOT FOR PRIMARY IMMUNISATIONS

CONSENT ~~DISC~~ WITH PARENTAL RESPONSIBILITY:

Measles	☐	Poliomyelitis	☐	Whooping Cough	☐
Mumps	☐	Diphtheria	☐	Hib	☐
Rubella	☐	Tetanus	☐		☐

~~sent to~~ ny ~~ch~~ d receiving these immunisations

Sig: ....   Date: ....

DELETE ANTIGENS NOT GIVEN

ANTIGEN	BATCH No.	DATE	ME		STAFF ID OR DESIGNATION
Measles					
Mumps					
Rubella					
BOOSTERS					
Diphtheria					
Tetanus					
Polio					
OTHER					
Hib					

Date and Result of any test of immunity for Rubella:

FP/73/2/GP (Revised 2/92)

Figure 9.11   Notification of immunisations of targeted children – FP73/2/GP.

Post-payment verification can be carried out both at the practice and at the HA.

HAs will use management information systems to enable them to undertake comparative analysis of claims against local and national averages. Claims may be investigated by routinely contacting patients, and at least once every three years practices will be visited by a team from the HA for an on-site verification of claims.

Practices should maintain up-to-date records in support of claims, and must make these records available as necessary to the verification teams. HA staff will need access to practice-held records to help with the verification of claims, and as this may include relevant entries in clinical records, it is important to ensure that confidentiality is maintained at all times.

How can practices prepare for verification visits?

- The health authority will normally contact the practice in advance to arrange a mutually suitable time for the visit.

- Normally the visit will be undertaken by two HA staff.

- Ensure *now* that you have adequate systems and records in place in support of claims, which are readily available for inspection. The HA will not impose systems on you, but you may wish to network with other local practices to share good practice in record keeping. A good audit trail will have source documents, dated and flagged with the identity of the person who created or updated them, stored in a form that can be readily accessed, and clearly traceable to claims.

- Ensure that your records are up to date.

- Ensure that you always obtain signatures where these are needed, or that you note clearly why they are not available.

- Ensure that staff who are preparing claims are competent in their preparation and are aware of the appropriate regulations.

- Note that the practice records accompanying the new forms do not constitute adequate evidence to support claims.

- Exploit your computer systems whenever possible to assist with the organisation of information.

- Test your systems regularly by tacking through random claims to see that the evidence is all available.

- HA staff will normally be seeking 100% verification. Ensure that you seek the same with your own checks.

- HA staff may be sampling 20 claims per claim type, and the visit may last approximately half a day per practice. A partner, or more likely the practice manager, should be available to assist with the process.

- Ensure that archived data are readily available. The sampled claims may stretch over a number of years.

- HA staff will discuss any findings with you before they leave. After the visit you will be sent a written report. If there are anomalies you may be invited to comment on the report before it is considered for action within the authority.

- Be prepared to raise any queries with HA staff. Regard this visit as an opportunity to improve working procedures and relationships.

Anomalies in claims would probably be detected by methods other than practice visits under most circumstances, so you should have been given an opportunity to sort these out. The visit is part of a verification process, not a check or formal audit. If for any reason you have concerns about a proposed visit, you should contact your local medical committee if you cannot resolve these concerns with the HA.

The following protocol is typical of the procedure adopted by health authorities when carrying out a post-payment verification visit.

Box 9.2 Post-payment verification (PPV) visit

1   **Post-payment verification visit objectives**

The general objective of PPV visits is for the health authority to gain assurance that claims submitted by practices are proper and in accordance with the Statement of Fees and Allowances (SFA). The visit is not exclusively looking for possible over-claims, but also for possible under-claims by practices. Specifically, the objectives are as follows:

- to gain assurance that GPs have provided the service to their patient for which claims for payment have been submitted to the health authority

- to assess whether claims made are in compliance with the SFA

- to disseminate good practice and to agree actions in respect of problem areas encountered

- to give the practice the opportunity to demonstrate their working practices and to raise any particular problems with which the PPV team could help.

2   **Composition of PPV visit**

Each practice visit will consist of two elements:

- an assessment of the control environment – to understand the systems and procedures within the practice for submitting each type of claim. This assessment will help to give assurance that claims are submitted properly and in accordance with the SFA

- a sample of claims paid will then be traced back to the underlying records to prove their validity.

3   **PPV visit method**

   3.1 Practice briefing

   An introductory briefing will take place at the start of the visit to discuss the format of the visit, the visit and practice roles and the likely time-scales expected for the visit.

3.2   Assessment of systems and procedures

An assessment of systems and procedures may highlight areas for improvement in controls over processing of claims, or in how to improve the efficiency of the way in which claims are processed (e.g. by reducing paperwork).

The objective of this assessment is to gain assurance that:

*   there are adequate procedures for recording services provided by the practice to patients

*   there is a satisfactory understanding and application of the provisions set out in the SFA in respect of each claim type

*   systems exist to prevent errors and omissions, as far as possible, in the claims submitted.

Discussions with practice staff will take place to establish the systems and procedures currently being used within the practice.

3.3   Items of service validation

3.3.1 Objective

The objective of this exercise is to ensure that all claims are valid (i.e. that they are in respect of treatment which took place). This is done by checking to see that each claim is supported by an appropriate entry in the practice records to prove that the patient was seen and received the treatment as claimed.

3.3.2 Sample selection

A random sample of claims received and paid by the health authority will be selected prior to attendance at the practice. The random sample will be taken from a range of claims which are normally submitted.

The sample size will be based on the list size of the practice in comparison with the average practice list size in the HA. The average list size per GP in most areas is 200, for which the sample size will be a total of 100 claims. The sample will be adjusted to reflect the list size of the practice being visited.

The claims selected will be validated against practice records.

3.3.3 *Access to medical records*

Access to patient medical records by the health authority visit team will be restricted to vouching for the specific medical entry in order to support the practice claim. The team will not require access, and should not request it, to other patient medical records.

The specific medical entry may be found by the practice manager or some other person nominated by the practice, and shown to the health authority team member.

Alternatively, to minimise the impact on the practice workload, the practice may prefer that the health authority staff find the relevant entries themselves. This is a matter of choice for the practice concerned and, where possible, their preference should be made known to the visit team in advance of the visit.

The procedure for accessing medical records is similar to that used by internal and external auditors at fundholding practices for the past five years.

All health authority and primary care trust staff are bound by their contractual obligations to maintain confidentiality at all times.

3.4 *Reporting*

At the completion stage of the post-payment verification practice visit, the visit team will give a verbal representation of the key findings of the visit. Practice verbal comments will be invited and documented.

A draft written report will be sent to practices for formal practice responses, which will be incorporated into the final report. The final report will then be sent to the practice.

Salaried general practitioners

Personal medical services (PMS)

Although many general practitioners like the autonomy of the 'independent contractor' status, there are some who prefer a regular structured income. The Primary Care Act of 1997 introduced salaried schemes for GPs, which are known as personal medical services (PMS). There are several pilot schemes in operation, including schemes involving NHS trusts and health authorities.

The NHS Plan encourages expansion of PMS contracts in England. With existing pilot schemes being made permanent, it is anticipated that by 2002 approximately one-third of GPs will work under this scheme.

10

Using information
technology

What's in the box: basic terminology

Box 10.1

Hardware	Physical components of the system, such as display screens, printers, keyboard, mouse, disks, etc.
Software	A set of programmed instructions in the computer which enable it to respond to input of information, and demands to change it, store it or print it out in various forms
CPU	The CPU, or central processor unit, is the part of the system that performs arithmetic operations and controls the storage, display, communication and manipulation of information. It is the part of the machine that is closest to a 'brain'
VDU	The screen that is used to display information held on the computer
Keyboard	A device like a typewriter for entering information into a computer. Many specialised systems use non-standard keyboards or make extensive use of special function keys to save typing effort
Mouse	A small hand-operated pointer which the user moves on a pad to move an arrow on the screen. Clicking a button on the mouse activates a number of operations without the need to type in text

Printer	A device that prints text and diagrams held on the computer on to paper. Older machines work like typewriters and are noisy and slow. Newer types work more like photocopiers or paint sprayers, and are much faster and quieter
Disk	Information cannot be permanently stored in the CPU. Usually it is stored on magnetic disk or tape. Tape is used for long-term secure storage and disks are used for information that is in constant use
Floppy disk	A disk which can be inserted into one computer and read by another. Most are 3.5 inches in diameter and contained in a rigid plastic case
Hard disk	A disk that is permanently held in the CPU and is used to store information needed on a permanent basis by a single user. Hard disks can hold many hundred times the information which can be stored by a floppy disk
Workstation	The work area where a computer operator works. Health and safety legislation gives details of how work-stations should be designed
Terminal	A machine that is capable of entering and retrieving information from a multi-user computer system. It may be a computer in its own right or, more usually, just a keyboard and screen
Network	When many people need to use the same computer system, several terminals can be linked together with cables. This, and the software needed for communication with a central CPU, is called a network
Byte	The measure of information that a computer can store. A byte is equivalent to a single text character, and one megabyte is equal to one million bytes. The more bytes of memory a computer or disk has, the more information it can store

How a computer works

It is not necessary to understand fully how computers work in order to operate the systems in use in GP practices, clinics and hospitals. The following brief outline is given merely for interest.

The central processor unit uses a system of on–off switches to hold information in a memory. Each number or character is expressed as a sequence of on or off states in a group of switches which together form a *byte*. As the operator enters information into the computer, it is translated into a machine-readable form and stored in the *random access memory* (RAM). This process is controlled by the computer's internal *operating system*. This is the raw material which is worked on by the computer's *application software*, which tells the machine how to display and manipulate the data to achieve the operator's needs, and how to interpret the instructions given by the operator.

The most common types of software are *word processors*, which enable the user to write documents, edit and print them. Most have facilities to store lists of names and addresses and insert these into one of a series of previously written standard letters. Routine correspondence can be produced far more efficiently in this way. Individual parts of a document can also be edited without the need for wholesale retyping. Importantly, information stored on one computer within a system (e.g. a patient administration system) can be imported on to another without the need to retype it.

Databases are applications designed to hold a lot of information about a series of people or things. An individual record (e.g. a patient) contains a variety of *fields* which may contain general text such as name, address and details of medical conditions. The field could have a specialised or limited range of values such as a postcode, date, or male or female, or it could be a code obtained from a published table such as diagnostic codings for different medical conditions. These codes are much easier for a computer system to analyse than is free text, which really needs a human brain to interpret it.

Spreadsheets are particularly suitable for arranging in order, displaying and performing calculations on mathematical data. They are commonly used to analyse treatments given to a large number of patients, or to calculate and report on budgets and expenditure. A typical small spreadsheet is shown in Table 10.1.

Table 10.1 Projected quarterly expenditure on staff training

Expenditure	First quarter	Second quarter	Third quarter	Fourth quarter
Staff time	£1287	£10 663	£7287	£5288
Expenses	£325	£8825	£8350	£3000
Total	£1612	£19 488	£15 637	£8288

Computers in general practice

General practice today is a highly complex organisation, and it is doubtful whether management of its administration can be effectively handled without information technology (IT). A computerised practice is:

- more efficient
- in greater control of patient care
- able to generate more income.

Patient benefits through computerisation

These include the following:

- improved preventive care through the identification of 'at-risk' groups, patient group analysis and follow-up
- reducing the risk of disease through immunisation/vaccination
- the early detection of disease through developmental screening, hypertensive monitoring, geriatric surveillance, etc.
- the management of established disease
- more selective advice on smoking, drinking, etc.
- better information on the patient services available.

The uses of an up-to-date patient database include the following:

- patient information data
- age–sex register
- logging and generation of repeat prescriptions
- logging and checking patient registration status
- checking immunisation/cervical cytology status
- screening and recall
- diagnosis and morbidity data
- opportunistic screening.

A computerised appointments system overcomes the difficulties of manual appointment books (e.g. illegible handwriting, pages messy with cancellations, two people not being able to use the book at the same time, handwritten surgery lists for pulling out records, are all circumvented).

Reference was made to using IT for written communication in Chapter 3. Secretaries and receptionists are now able to produce letters using a word-processing package to generate mailmerged letters, or readily produce letters to patients. Spreadsheets can be used either to collect data (for display in tables, graphs and pie charts) or to present doctor and staff rotas.

Desktop publishing software can be used to generate leaflets, posters and handouts.

Technology can save time for some tasks. For others it does not save time, but it does make it possible to produce professional-looking documents (e.g. practice leaflets, charts and posters).

For those who enjoy using a computer, it is essential that the computer does not become a barrier between the patient and the secretary or receptionist. Remember that it is as rude to continue to input or extract data as it is to continue to talk to a colleague or take a telephone call without acknowledging the presence of a patient.

The major disadvantage of IT in the practice is when the system 'goes down'. The increased efficiency then disappears and returning to manual systems, no matter how temporarily, results in unavoidable delays and disruption.

Age–sex register and patient information

These are basic patient data which are put on to the computer. Secretaries and receptionists will receive specific training in the use of their practice's information system.

The importance of inputting data accurately cannot be overstated, as this information will be of vital importance to the practice's activities. Remember, too, always to include the postcode. This is a vital piece of information and it should be cross-checked with the medical record in your possession.

You should be aware of the requirements of the Data Protection Act, and you must respect the security and confidentiality of patient information at all times.

Registration data

This data is of immense value. It includes the following information about registration status:

- the date on which the patient was registered with the practice
- the date on which the patient was accepted onto the doctor's list
- the date on which the patient was included on a GP's patient list.

It will also indicate the category and date of a patient's removal from a doctor's list (e.g. when moving out of the area, or on death).

Repeat prescriptions

A computerised system can save much of the receptionist's time by obviating the need to retrieve patient files and other manually held prescribing information. In addition:

- it produces a legible, printed and accurate prescription
- it places a time limit on the issue of repeat prescriptions
- it monitors the rate and consumption of drugs
- it updates the repeat prescription record
- it easily identifies patients who are on a particular medication.

Screening and recall

The ability of a computer to search rapidly on the basis of specific criteria can allow a practice to identify certain groups of patients, including:

- those selected for information (e.g. asthmatics, hypertensives, diabetics, etc.) for health-promotion banding, and who would benefit from additional care and those who are considered to be 'at risk'
- those who are eligible for item-of-service claims.

The computer can also help with the following:

- crisis intervention
- the control of chronic diseases
- preventive medicine
- generating additional income for the practice.

Diagnoses and morbidity

A computer has the capacity and speed to extract and analyse data on any topics of particular interest to the practice (e.g. to analyse morbidity and treatment within the practice). The latest Royal College of General Practitioners (RCGP) coding system has been developed with a view to collecting these types of data from as many practices as possible.

Social recording

Computer systems are also capable of recording information on height/weight/smoking and alcohol-related habits in order to provide the health authority/health board with statistics for practices claiming health-promotion banding allowances. This information is automatically included in the patients' records.

Electronic links and other developments

Information technology is rapidly advancing, and over 7000 medical practices are now linked directly to health authorities across England and Wales. All health authorities and trusts are now transmitting items of service to over 3000 practices.

Electronic links convey correspondence, such as patient test results and consultant letters, directly between the sender's and the recipient's computer systems. The electronic linkage is made by using public and private telephone networks. The technical term used for the transfer of such data is electronic data interchange (EDI), where the sender's information is converted into a form which can be conveyed through telephone lines via a modem.

The advantages of electronic links are as follows:

- less duplication of tasks (e.g. patient registration)
- fewer transcription errors (where data are entered only once)
- reduced paperwork (form-filling)
- easier and faster access to information.

The main applications of electronic links are as follows:

- links with the practice health authority for the exchange of:

- patient registration information
- items-of-service claims
• links with local hospitals for the exchange of:
    - patient referral correspondence between GPs and consultants
    - laboratory test results and reports and requests from GPs.

Pathology links are being used by health authorities and trusts to facilitate the transmission of results of tests to general medical practitioners. The main benefit of this is that individual test results (e.g. blood haemoglobin level or results of a full blood count) can be 'posted' directly into the

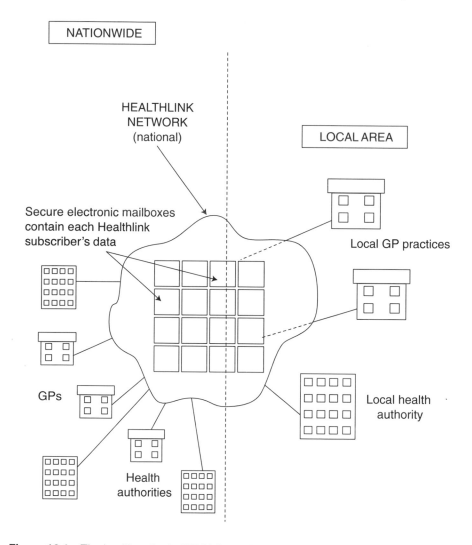

Figure 10.1   The health authority/GP Links project: making the connections.

clinical notes of patients. 'Posting' avoids the need to type the results into the system, thereby saving time and possible data-entry errors. Doctors will be able to select which results they wish to see (e.g. abnormal results highlighted by the laboratory will be displayed on the screen).

As well as being 'posted' into the notes, results may also be marked 'for action' by practice staff (e.g. a re-test or an appointment with the GP may be necessary).

As part of the *Patients Not Paper* initiative, the NHS Executive has set up a project called GP Provider Links ('Trailblazers'), which is pioneering standard communication links between practices and hospitals. *See* Figure 10.1.

Electronic medicine: what is happening now?

Technology is advancing so rapidly in the health service that it is difficult to keep up to date with exactly what is going on. You will have found that in the workplace your computers are being used increasingly for recording of data, and that they are linked to your health authority or trust. The terms 'NHSnet', 'LINKS' and 'telemedicine' are now commonplace.

Box 10.2 More computer 'jargon'

Internet	A framework which allows the exchange of information between computers
Internet provider	A company which provides access to the Internet. There are a number of providers and a choice of ways to pay for the connection
Website	A source of information on the Internet on many topics and subjects, arranged on individual pages
Network interface	The part of the computer that enables information to be transmitted over a telephone line
Modem	Hardware that allows the computer to 'talk' over a telephone line. It may be used as a network interface

NHSnet

This is the NHS's private Internet, which aims to bring about fast and easy access to vital information through the convergence of the Internet and e-health. So much is happening at the present time, with various schemes being piloted, that it is difficult to keep abreast of current developments. We may rest assured that measures are being taken to implement electronic healthcare. The NHS Plan states that the NHS will have the most up-to-date information technology systems to deliver services for patients more rapidly and more conveniently, with many millions of pounds being invested in modernising IT systems.

In previous chapers it has been seen that information technology is already linking primary and secondary care services. It is possible for patients to consult their GP via the Internet, and consultants and GPs may run Internet-linked clinics with one another. Patients may be able to call at the surgery and consult a specialist from a local hospital. It is all happening now! The NHS Plan also states that all GP practices will be connected to the NHSnet by 2002, giving patients improved diagnosis, information and referral.

It is possible for doctors all over the world to communicate via the Internet, which is able to access vast amounts of information, websites on individual health, and research databases such as *Medline* (which provides details of medical articles published worldwide).

What e-health will do

With the reality of e-health dawning, patients and healthcare professionals should all see an improved and more responsive service that brings about fast and easy access to vital information.

NHS Direct online

NHS Direct online is the gateway to health advice and information on the Internet. It includes an easy-to-use guide to treating common symptoms at home, and links to thousands of sources of help and advice.

National Electronic Library for Health (NeLH)

NeLH is a new NHS website for health professionals, providing up-to-date best practice information on diagnosis and treatment.

Telemedicine Information Service

The Telemedicine Information Service provides a directory giving details of and contacts for around 120 UK telemedicine projects. This service is provided by the British Library in conjunction with a healthcare computing group. Individuals who do not have access to the Internet can interrogate the database by telephone.

Electronic health records (EHR)

By 2004 it is anticipated that more than 50% of hospitals, as well as primary and community trusts, will have implemented electronic patient record systems. The EHR aims to build a lifetime electronic health record for all citizens, which is able to be accessed from all parts of the UK and ultimately worldwide. This will mean that patients' healthcare records are accessible by all stakeholders, including social care professionals, whenever and wherever they may be needed. A project such as this is a vast undertaking that requires careful planning to implement an integrated system.

Telemedicine

Telemedicine is the term given to electronic means of delivering health services. It allows doctors many miles apart to communicate both with one another and with patients, and to conduct live consultations from all over the world via the Internet. By adding a camera to the system, video conferencing or video telemedicine becomes possible, whereby all parties involved can view each other, thus simulating a 'live' consultation.

There are certain areas where telemedicine could be particularly useful, such as the treatment of terminally ill patients at home. Videophones would enable patients, carers or relatives to communicate with clinicians without having to make the journey to hospital. Telemedicine could also be useful for supporting medical staff in crisis situations, enabling them to obtain expert advice from remote links.

Future implementation plans

The NHS information strategy stipulates that all trusts should have electronic prescribing systems in place by 2005, which will help to prevent the types of errors that may occur with handwritten prescriptions in hospitals.

New technology will enable cross-matching of blood samples to be performed electronically, thereby saving staff time and money, as well as facilitating the provision of blood for trauma victims. Hospital laboratories are being given the go-ahead to move towards electronic cross-matching (EXR).

Computers in hospitals

Computerisation of records in hospitals works well because there is a great deal of information to be stored and consulted, information is required by a variety of people at different times and in different locations, much of the information needs to be sorted or changed, and complex analysis of data is required.

This is not because computers are 'clever'. They are not – they have no real intelligence or ability to think of solutions. However, computers can process vast amounts of data at incredible speed with virtually no errors. A 'computer error' is almost always due to a human operator doing the wrong thing or the computer's programmer setting it up wrongly in the first place.

The main systems used in hospitals are the patient administration system (PAS), word processing, and record storage in pathology, X-ray and pharmacy departments. Other major systems are used in finance and personnel departments, estates management and supplies, and are being introduced into nursing and theatre management.

Patient administration systems (PAS)

The potential of computers has long been exploited in hospitals in the area of patient administration. There are many versions used by different hospitals, but all of them have the same component parts (*see* Box 10.3).

Box 10.3

Patient index	Records of the personal details of every patient
Admissions, discharges and transfers	A record of each patient's history of time spent in the hospital as an inpatient or outpatient, with particular consultants or in a particular department
Waiting-lists	Names and dates of referral of all patients waiting for inpatient and/or outpatient treatment
Outpatients	A system to manage appointments and correspondence associated with outpatient clinics
GP index	A list of the names and addresses of all of the local GPs

Nursing management systems

Increasingly, hospitals are being equipped with computer systems to help nurses to plan and keep track of the nursing care of patients. Patients' details are retrieved from **PAS**, and a detailed plan of their expected care is prepared. Care given is recorded on the system to help to co-ordinate the work of the team. Patient dependency levels can be predicted from the care plans, and nurse rosters are drawn up to match needs.

Order communication systems

In most hospitals, ordering portering services, pathology tests, supplies of materials or repairs to buildings or equipment must be done by telephone or by completing a form, often with multiple copies and requiring posting to the relevant department. This can take a long time and involve much duplication of effort. An order communications (or 'order-comms') system allows ordering departments to send requests for services directly to the department, and to receive confirmation of orders or the results of tests directly.

Hospital information support system (HISS)

The trend among hospitals with well-established computer systems is to integrate them into one powerful scheme called a hospital information support system (HISS). Such a system allows every department's computer system to communicate with those of other departments, to transfer information and to generate reports.

Information, management and technology

Implementing *Information for Health* (IfH)

Implementing *Information for Health* is a national priority for the NHS and an important programme underpinning the Modernisation Agenda (*see* Chapter 1). The main targets for *Information for Health* are described below.

Targets to be achieved by the end of 2002 are as follows:

- 35% of all acute hospitals to have implemented a Level 3 electronic patient record (EPR)

- substantial progress in implementing integrated primary care and community EPRs in 25% of health authorities

- NHSnet to be used for appointments booking, referrals, radiology and laboratory requests/results in all parts of the country

- community prescribing with electronic links to GPs and the Prescription Pricing Authority

- telemedicine and telecare options considered routinely in all health improvements programmes

- a national electronic library for health, accessible through local 'intranets' in all NHS organisations

- information strategies as appropriate to underpin completed National Service Frameworks

- beacon electronic health record (EHR) sites.

Targets to be achieved by 2005 are as follows:

- full implementation at primary care level of first-generation person-based EHR

- all acute hospitals with Level 3 EHR

- electronic transfer of patient records between GPs

- 24-hour emergency access to patient records.

IfH is part of the wide government agenda that is aiming to:

- build services around citizens' choice

- make Government and its services more accessible

- improve social inclusion

- use information more effectively to improve services and achieve targets

IfH was published in 1998. Its key elements are as follows:

- lifelong electronic health records for every person in the country

- round-the-clock online access to patient records, and information about best clinical practice, for all NHS clinicians

- genuinely seamless care for patients through GPs, hospitals and community services sharing information across the NHS information highway

- fast and convenient public access to online information and care.

Box 10.4   Some useful acronyms

CHDGP	Collecting Health Data from General Practice
CTI	Computers in Teaching Initiative
EHR	Electronic Health Record
IM&T	Information, Management and Technology
LIS	Local Implementation Strategy
NeLH	National Electronic Library for Health
RHI	Regional Head of Information
RFA	Requirements for Accreditation of GP Systems

Getting the best from the computer

The importance of inputting data accurately cannot be overstated, as this information is to be used by healthcare professionals when treating and caring for patients, and for statistical analysis and planning, budgeting, contract monitoring and invoicing for services. Information held on the computer must be regularly cross-checked with that held on medical records, and it should be amended as necessary. Incorrect information about a patient can lead to important letters or test results going astray.

Problems which arise in hospitals are frequently caused by out-of-date addresses, either because the patient has moved house or changed GP, or both. Other problems arise from incomplete details, or temporary addresses entered as permanent ones (e.g. when a person is taken ill when visiting relatives). Errors in this information can be very costly to the hospital, since if the bill is sent to the wrong health authority or GP fundholder, they are unlikely to pay.

The barrier created by the computer

Computer systems usually require the input of patient information in a specific sequence, which may not be the same as that which the patient wants to give. Sometimes the computer is slow to respond if many people are using it. Receptionist staff frequently have to deal with a patient on the telephone, another in person, and call up details on to their screen, all at the same time. Both the patient and the receptionist may start to feel that they are the servant of the computer, rather than the other way round.

To overcome these difficulties it is important to explain to the patient what is happening (especially when you are on the telephone), and to develop a sequence of questions which gives the information you need in the correct order. This often requires a good deal of practice and discussion with colleagues before it works really well.

Maintaining security

There are four main risks to be guarded against when using computer systems:

* unauthorised access to information held on computer

* loss of information due to mechanical failure

* theft of machinery

* spoiling of information by computer viruses.

Preventing unauthorised access

Information about people that is held on computer is governed by the Data Protection Act. It should only be used for the purpose for which it was collected and should not be revealed to unauthorised individuals. Where password systems exist, these must be used, and passwords should never be shared or revealed to others. Computer screens should face away from public areas. Terminals should not be left unattended showing data or even 'logged on' to a system, since anyone may then gain access.

Backing up – keeping spare copies of information

If information has been stored on a computer's hard disk and it is lost due to mechanical failure or theft, a great deal of work will be needed to replace it. It is therefore extremely important to keep copies on a separate storage device. Taking such copies is known as *backing up,* and should be done daily. Staff using a multi-user system may find that this is done centrally by a system manager. Each night the latest data is copied on to large tape recorders.

Personal computers should be backed up either to a central back-up store via a hospital network, or to removable floppy disks or specially designed tape records (called tape streamers). Locally made back-up copies should be stored away from the computer in case of theft or fire.

Guarding against theft

Backing up is also important in case a computer is stolen. Such thefts from hospitals and healthcare premises are becoming increasingly common. All premises should be secure and kept locked. Machinery should be indelibly marked and preferably fastened to the desktop and alarmed with one of a variety of proprietary products. Computers should be housed away from public view wherever possible (e.g. away from windows without blinds).

Computer viruses

These are small programs designed to damage data that is held on computer. They are transferred from one machine to another when other files are copied, perhaps from floppy disk or by electronic connection. To guard against this, material should never be copied from a disk which has not been checked for viruses, nor should games and other such programs be copied on to work machines. Computer equipment and disks should be routinely checked for the presence of virus programs.

Illegal use of software

Commercial computer programs are protected by copyright. In general, a program can only be used on one computer unless a site licence has been purchased. The penalties for using programs which are not licensed are extremely high.

Computers and the law

Where medical records are stored on computer it is a requirement that computer-held material is at least as confidential as a paper record. Special care must be taken with computerised information, since it is possible to write programs which allow different people different levels of access. For example, it is possible to give a doctor access via the computer to all of the information that is held, whereas the clerk may only see certain material. Some staff will be allowed to change information, while others will have 'read only' access.

Data protection (*see* Chapter 4)

Organisations which record information on computer relating to identifiable living individuals must ensure that they comply with the provisions of the Data Protection Act. This Act applies to England, Wales, Scotland and Northern Ireland.

The Data Protection Act is based on eight principles, and is designed to ensure that information relating to an individual is obtained fairly, is kept up to date and is stored securely. The individual whose data are stored has rights of access enabling him or her to check the accuracy of the information. The data protection registrar and the courts are empowered to require correction of inaccurate material if it is not undertaken voluntarily by the data user.

New developments

The aim of the NHS information strategy is to ensure that data can move securely throughout the NHS network. For example:

- requirements for accreditation are intended to develop a convergence of system standards, thus simplifying the task of enabling computer systems to communicate with each other

- new NHS numbers will avoid the problems of number duplication and simplify patient confidentiality with EDI

- an NHS network will consist of a national network linking all health authorities and central registries, to which will be linked local networks to include laboratories, hospitals and GP surgeries.

Looking forward: the computer-based patient record

The electronic patient record in the UK

In January 1994, the Information Management Group of the NHS Executive organised a three-year project to enable healthcare professionals in acute hospitals to give better care to patients through the use of the electronic patient records systems. The outcome of the research is intended to feed into the development of clinical systems which will be available at some point in the future. A major objective is to improve patient care through electronic patient record systems and to explore the value to clinicians of integrated electronic patient record systems. The following reasons for developing the computerised patient record were outlined in *Aspects of the Computer-based Patient Record* (1992):

- the uses of and demand for patient data are increasing

- the increasing complexity of treatments and an increasing elderly population

- a mobile population which needs to be tracked

- to improve quality and manage costs.

Electronic patient records (EPR) can include everything that is currently held in the paper record, and may contain text, sound and images (e.g. X-rays). The information contained in the EPR can be sorted, summarised or reported on and put to a number of uses.

Patient administration systems used in hospitals contain mostly administrative details, but there are also the much larger hospital information support systems (HISS). These contain many patient-based details, including order communications and incorporated test results.

Another type of electronic record is known as the 'smart card' (similar to the plastic credit card), which has information recorded on an integrated circuit chip. These cards contain the patient's identification details, blood groups, allergies, GP and a summary of their medical record. The benefits of smart cards are that they are portable and can be held by patients.

There are no examples in the UK as yet of a fully integrated EPR system, although some hospitals are working towards fully computerised records.

The new NHS number

The key to effective sharing of information about patients is the ability to identify a person in a way which is common throughout the NHS. The use of a common single identifier will be the key to the exchange of clinical and administrative information between systems and healthcare workers. The existing NHS number is not suitable for computerised information systems and will in due course be replaced.

The 'paperless' practice

It has been suggested that medical practices should become 'paperless'. Indeed, many practices would like to take advantage of computerised record keeping and electronic transfer of data, as this would lead to a reduction in practice workload and ensure legibility and uniformity of medical records. Unfortunately, current systems are not designed to produce a literary patient record, but they do provide an excellent record of drug history and details of current treatment.

The GP's terms of service do not recognise computer records, and it is therefore possible that a paperless practice could be found to be in breach of its terms of service. Although some practices do keep computerised records, they maintain paper records at the same time. There is no doubt that, in the future, legitimate computerised medical records will be possible, but only when a suitable system has been developed through which full medical records can be transferred electronicallly between different areas of the health service.

GP links to the NHSnet

Patients in the community will benefit from the connection of every GP surgery and hospital to the NHSnet (e.g. due to quicker results, on-line specialist advice and ease of appointments). Demonstration sites are planned, and these services will be available across the UK by 2002.

11

Medical terminology and clinical aspects

Introduction

Medical secretaries and receptionists, with their unique skills in dealing with doctors, other professionals and patients with tact and courtesy, will find that a knowledge of medical terminology will help them to carry out their duties in a more effective and efficient manner. Very often the words and phrases used by medical professionals are long, difficult and apparently obscure.

Medical terminology is based upon root words derived from Greek and Latin. To these roots may be added syllables that modify the meaning of the root word. An addition made to the front of a root is known as a *prefix*, and an addition at the end is known as a *suffix*. Over the years this principle has been modified in such a way that it can be applied to modern medical techniques. For example, the word 'gaster' (Greek) means 'stomach'. The root word used in medical terminology is 'gastr-o' and by adding the suffix 'itis', the word is modified to *gastritis*, meaning 'inflammation of the stomach'. By adding the suffix 'oscopy', we obtain the word *gastroscopy*, which means in this modified form 'visual inspection of the stomach' (by means of a gastroscope).

It is not intended to go into a detailed explanation of medical terminology here, but rather to point out that a limited knowledge of some root words, prefixes and suffixes will give a wider understanding of the medical vocabulary. Appendix 4 lists some of the most commonly used root words, prefixes and suffixes.

Medical abbreviations are also frequently used by professionals in healthcare, and again a knowledge of these will be of value (*see* Appendix 4).

Pathology and X-ray examinations

Medical secretaries and receptionists will find that doctors refer patients for pathological and other investigations and tests. An awareness of the most commonly used tests will not only contribute to the effectiveness of their day-to-day work, but will also make their job more interesting and fulfilling (*see* Appendix 4).

Prescribing and drugs

The supply, distribution and storage of drugs are controlled by a series of Acts of Parliament which are designed to control their sale and reduce their danger to life from sale by unqualified individuals.

Secretaries and receptionists will find that a knowledge of the drugs most frequently used by the medical practice or hospital consultant will be of value in their day-to-day work.

Receptionists in general practice have greater direct involvement with repeat prescribing for their patients, and will often have to deal with queries. However, the receptionist must have clear instructions and never be placed in the position of having to make medical decisions.

Components of a prescription

The following information must be included on every prescription issued by the doctor, whether it is an NHS or private prescription. Without this information it is not possible for the pharmacist to dispense the drugs. Sometimes the writing on the prescription may be illegible, but this is not so common now that repeat prescriptions in general practice are computer generated.

Drug name

This may be written as the generic or approved name of the drug, or its trade or proprietary name. For example:

- salbutamol (generic)
- Ventolin (proprietary).

Form of prescribed drug

This refers to whether capsules, tablets, syrup, injection, ointment, etc. are required.

Strength

Many drugs are available in more than one strength, which must be specified.

Directions

Directions to the patient regarding the dosage of the medicine should be included. The *British National Formulary* recommends that directions should preferably be written in English. However, some doctors still use Latin abbreviations (*see* Appendix 4).

Amount or quantity

A box on the prescription form can be completed to indicate the number of days for which the treatment is to continue. If this is not used, the quantity to be dispensed should be included.

Problems with prescriptions

Medical receptionists and secretaries should be aware that problems can be caused by the following:

- missing information (e.g. strength of drug, missing form or type of drug, missing dose)
- incorrect or inaccurate information (e.g. incorrect name of drug) (similar drug names can cause problems – for instance, *chlorpropamide* which is used for treating diabetes and *chlorpromazine*, an antipsychotic drug)
- incorrect strength or incorrect dose
- amounts of medicine prescribed (patients often complain that they have run out of one medicine and still have some others left. Remember that medicines come in different pack sizes – some in 28s, some in 30s, etc.).

Controlled drugs

The relevant legislation concerning controlled drugs is the Misuse of Drugs Regulations 1985 and subsequent amendments.

For controlled drugs there are rules for the following:

- who can possess and supply
- record keeping
- storage
- prescription writing.

Records

Secretaries and receptionists should understand that it is the doctor's duty to maintain a register, in an approved form, of the quantity of all controlled drugs obtained and supplied, including any administered personally, with names and addresses.

Storage

All controlled drugs in the custody of a doctor must be kept in a locked cupboard that can only be opened by the doctor or with his or her authority.

It is the doctor's responsibility to ensure that the controlled drugs cupboard is locked and the keys put safely away. The medical secretary or receptionist should make sure that this has been done.

Prescribing controlled drugs

Special rules apply to the prescribing of controlled drugs. A prescription for a controlled drug must:

- be written in ink, or otherwise so as to be indelible, and it must be signed and dated by the person issuing it with his or her usual signature
- be written by the person issuing it in his or her own handwriting
- specify the name and address of the person for whom it is intended
- specify the strength of the preparation, the dose to be taken and the quantity of the preparation in both words and figures.

An exception to these rules is phenobarbitone. Receptionists can write prescriptions for this, but the quantity must be written in both words and figures.

Some general medical practitioners in England and Wales use a special prescription form (FP10 (MDA)) for treatment of addicts by instalment with the controlled drug *methadone*.

Only medical practitioners who hold a special licence from the Home Secretary can prescribe the controlled drugs *cocaine*, *diamorphine* and *dipipanone* for addiction, although all general medical practitioners can still prescribe these drugs for relief of pain due to illness or injury, without a special licence.

Repeat prescribing

The doctor is responsible for issuing the initial prescription to the patient, and for explaining what the preparation is and what it is intended to do, etc. The patient does not always remember this information, and will often discuss any problems with the receptionist or secretary.

Some patients are on regular drug regimes and are able to request repeat prescriptions without seeing the doctor every time they run out of their medication.

In general practice, receptionists play a vital role in the repeat prescription procedure of the practice.

- They receive the requests from patients for a repeat of their medication.

- They will either prepare a further prescription for the doctor's signature, or generate a repeat prescription on the practice computer to be signed by the doctor.

- A record should be kept either on the computer or in the patient's medical record (or both) of repeat prescribing.

- They will explain to the patient how to make the best use of the repeat prescription service offered by the practice (e.g. the procedures and system used – the use of cards, computer printout, or telephone requests for repeat prescriptions).

The repeat prescription system used by the medical practice is designed not only to make better use of the doctor's time, but also to suit the patient's needs. Every practice has its own system to ensure that patients obtain their prescriptions on a regular basis.

Many pharmacies now offer a repeat medication service which is operated in co-operation with local medical practices. Patients or carers who wish to take advantage of such a service must initiate requests for their repeat prescriptions to be directed to a particular pharmacy for dispensing. Reception staff are often responsible for placing these repeat prescriptions in bags provided by local pharmacies, which are collected on a regular basis by pharmacy employees. The ready-dispensed prescriptions are then collected by patients from the respective pharmacy, or are delivered to the housebound by arrangement. The role of the receptionist is very important for the smooth running of 'collection and delivery' repeat medication services.

Computer-generated prescriptions

Many practices now have a computer which will generate repeat prescriptions, instead of receptionists having to laboriously write them out. Although computer-generated prescriptions are time saving, secretaries and receptionists must remember that computers are only efficient if the correct information has been entered in the first place. Therefore, when entering details of patients' medication into the computer, always check that all of the information is there (e.g. that the right drug, its strength, the correct dose and quantity have been entered).

The same attention to detail is necessary when making amendments to existing drug records – for example, when doses have been changed following a clinical review of the patient and their medication by the medical practitioner. It is therefore extremely important that computer records are kept up to date with accurate data.

Sources of information

Doctors receive a great deal of information which is designed to help them when prescribing for their patients. Medical secretaries and receptionists will no doubt have access to the following useful sources of information:

*   the *British National Formulary* (*BNF*)

*   the *Monthly Index of Medical Specialities* (*MIMS*).

The *BNF*, which is published twice yearly, is an official and reliable source of accurate information on prescribing. *MIMS* is sent to doctors each month. It is a good, 'user-friendly' information source, but printing errors may occasionally occur. Both publications provide details of constituents, manufacturers, packaging, net costs, etc., of every medicine that can be prescribed.

Branded or generic

Every drug that a doctor prescribes will fall into one of two categories:

* branded
* generic.

The term 'branded' refers to the proprietary name of a drug that is given by a manufacturer, whilst the term 'generic' means that the name is a general one which describes the pharmacological product. Both the *BNF* and *MIMS* give cross-referenced information on generic and brand-named products.

There is an increasing trend for medical practitioners to prescribe generic drugs, as they are often cheaper than their 'branded' or proprietary equivalents. Sometimes, as a result of practice policy, patients on repeat medication are 'switched' to generic drugs and need reassurance that their new medication has essentially the same action as the original 'branded' medication.

Practice prescribing policies

Prescribing analyses and costs (PACT)

Secretaries and receptionists in general practice will be aware that their practice prescribing policy to a certain extent reflects national and local guidelines.

The Prescription Pricing Authority (PPA) sends a statement each quarter giving information on what individual doctors and the whole practice are prescribing, how much is being spent on drugs, and how they compare locally and nationally with other doctors and practices. Health authorities indicate a target cost for each practice to aim for, which is designed to encourage effective prescribing procedures. The local primary care group or trust, through its prescribing subcommittee or the equivalent, generates guidance for practices on prescribing, which also reflects the needs of the local population.

Practice formularies

There are many medicines and preparations available on prescription, a number of which are the same generic drug with a different proprietary name. Practices are reducing the number of drugs they prescribe and, where appropriate yet in the patient's best interests, will try to achieve the national approach.

The community pharmacist

Pharmacists, in common with general practitioners, have a contract with the NHS which clearly states their terms of service. This contract, together with the requirements of the Medicines Act, provides the framework within which pharmacists work.

The pharmacist is a professional person who will from time to time telephone a medical practice to speak to a doctor or a member of the team. This may be to query a prescription item or the frequency of its repeat. The receptionist or secretary should always immediately connect the pharmacist to the doctor, being aware that they are acting in accordance with legal and professional responsibility.

Many community pharmacists keep computerised records of medicines dispensed to patients, and are thus readily aware of potential problems.

A recent development has been the introduction of 'primary care pharmacists' who are based in medical practices. They are often community pharmacists whose roles involve supporting the practice in achieving rational and cost-effective prescribing, for example by:

- advising on repeat-prescribing policies

- reviewing medication changes on patients' discharge from hospital

- assisting with the development of practice formularies.

Medicines management

Recent initiatives involving the pharmacy profession have been associated with implementing the government's NHS Plan. All are based around meeting the changing needs of patients.

A number of community pharmacists have become involved in locally or nationally organised *medicines management* projects. The goal of medicines management is to optimise prescribing and help patients who need it to make better use of their medicines. Pharmacists are using their skills as part of multidisciplinary teams, introducing an intervention process into the relationship between the community pharmacist, the patient and the GP. For example, in collaboration with GP practices, pharmacists are helping to target patients with coronary heart disease, following NSF guidance. Selected patients are interviewed, their medication reviewed, adverse drug effects identified and compliance issues addressed. It is anticipated that all PCTs will have medicines management initiatives by 2004.

Repeat dispensing schemes have been initiated to allow patients to obtain prescriptions from their GPs, which can then be dispensed by their pharmacists in several instalments. When patients, many with chronic conditions, collect their instalments, pharmacists have an opportunity to confirm that the prescription still meets their needs. These schemes have proved convenient for patients and waste of medicines has been reduced. Repeat dispensing schemes will be in place nationwide by 2004.

The *electronic transmission of prescriptions* is undergoing NHS trials. NHS-wide standards will be developed to allow routine electronic transfer of prescriptions in the community as well as hospitals. Patients should benefit from easier ordering of repeat prescriptions while pharmacists will benefit from the new opportunities to use information technology to support their practice.

E-pharmacy developments allow people to consult their pharmacist electronically to seek advice, purchase over-the-counter medicines, and to make arrangements for the delivery of their dispensed prescriptions. In due course, the introduction of electronic prescribing is likely to mean that a prescription could be transferred to a pharmacy electronically, thereby widening the dispensing choice available to patients.

Finally, *extending prescribing rights to pharmacists* is likely to build upon the success of nurse prescribing. Following new legislation, extension will begin with 'supplementary prescribing', when suitably qualified pharmacists will be responsible for the continuing care of patients who have been clinically assessed by an independent prescriber. *Pharmacist prescribing* might include pharmacists' involvement in anti-coagulant clinics, where treatment requires careful monitoring and adjustment of doses. Adding a prescribing role to existing responsibilities will enable pharmacists to provide a better and more efficient service for patients.

12

Primary healthcare services and social services

Introduction

The government's policy in recent years has been to transfer care from the secondary to the primary sector – that is, from hospitals or other institutions (such as long-term inpatient psychiatric care) to the patients being cared for at home and supported there by relevant services.

These policies are embodied in the *Health of the Nation* documents which set out health targets for the nation. Within local settings, for example in Wales, health authorities/health boards have set out local strategies for health aligned with the *Health of the Nation* strategy, but breaking it down into achievable aims and objectives at the local level. The Community Care Act supplements the *Health of the Nation* strategy by providing a structure to manage the patients in their own homes.

The Community Care Act gives patients (or clients) an active part in deciding what care they receive, compared with the previous situation where the health authority and social services provided a range of services and the patient received the service deemed to be most appropriate for them by doctors, nurses or social workers.

Care in the community includes both community nursing services and social services. As each patient is referred to the community nursing services (from a hospital, a general practitioner or by self-referral), an assessment is conducted with the patient, and with their relatives if they wish, in the home. A nursing care plan is agreed which is tailored to meet the needs of the patient. Typical services provided by community nurses would include giving injections (e.g. insulin to housebound diabetics), palliative care to patients who are dying, and dressings and removal of stitches after surgery. Patients do not make any personal contribution to the cost of their care (i.e. the service is free).

With social services, a care plan is agreed between the patient and the social worker. However, the patient's financial situation is also taken into account in order to work out the patient's contribution towards the cost. (Patients have made a contribution towards social services received for some time, and no one goes without a service they need simply because they cannot afford it.) Social services provide for children and families, the elderly, and patients with mental illness, learning difficulties, permanent disabilities and alcohol problems. To supplement care given by families, friends and neighbours, help may come from the following sources:

- social workers, home carers and meals on wheels

- sheltered housing, day centres, residential homes and nursing homes

- wardens and housing officers

- voluntary groups, visitors and churches.

Apart from meals on wheels, which delivers a hot cooked meal to the patient's home, luncheon clubs encourage patients to socialise, carer support groups encourage family members and friends to share their experiences and support one another, and information services help patients and families to know what is available to them. Simple practical help, such as assistance with bathing, light housework or preparing a meal, is now provided by home carers who are specially trained to do this work.

Further information about community nursing or social services provided in any particular area of the country will be available from local offices who publish leaflets outlining what they provide, to whom, and how to access the services.

The limit on funds for health and social care results in decisions being made about what service or care is received dependent on funds available. This concept is very difficult for a nation that has come to depend on a free health service which is available to all at the point of need. The reality of the situation is that the Government does not have a bottomless purse, so the responsibility for deciding who receives what care is being transferred to those who deal with the patients – doctors and health and social care workers. Therefore the role of health professionals is changing from 'helping people' and responding to need, to include assessment and management, and offsetting need against available funds.

Dentists, opticians and pharmacists, like general practitioners, are contracted to the health authorities to provide their services. They are also greatly affected by the changes to the funding and structure of the health service. Fewer dental and optical services are available to patients on the

NHS, so their NHS income has dropped. To remain viable, they charge patients for services and sell related products, or become entirely private practice. Pharmacists' income is directly related to the value of prescriptions dispensed. Doctors are reducing their prescription bills to meet their indicative prescribing budgets, so pharmacists' income is also decreasing. They supplement their income by selling more 'over-the-counter' and associated products, and some independent local chemists are being taken over by larger chains.

The NHS Plan indicates that a new level of primary care trust is being established which will commission both health and social services in one package, thus ensuring, well-integrated 'seamless' healthcare.

Trusts and fundholding

The White Paper *Working for Patients* led to the reforms stated in the NHS and Community Care Act 1990, such as the 'internal market', where 'providers' of healthcare (hospitals, community services and ambulances) were separated from 'purchasers' (GPs and local health authorities). Purchasers were given a budget to enable them to purchase services from the providers.

This led to the emergence of NHS trusts, which enabled providers to be independent, self-managed, competitive providers of healthcare in the internal market. General medical practices were given the opportunity to become 'fundholders', where they had the freedom to purchase healthcare which would best fulfil the needs of their patients. A budget was allocated to give GPs this freedom of choice in the best interests of patients.

Approximately 50% of GP practices had become fundholding practices, but with a change of Government, and the Health Act of 1999, GP fundholding was abolished. The main reason for ending fundholding was that it was felt that the NHS had become a 'two-tiered' system, with patients from fundholding practices being able to obtain secondary healthcare and treatment more quickly than patients from non-fundholder practices.

Fundholding has not been abolished in Northern Ireland, and indeed there has been considerable further expansion.

By 1995, trust status had been given to ambulance services. Their whole range of services, from transporting patients to hospital outpatient clinics, to emergency admissions, doctors' answering service, paging, community alarms and nursing answering service are now managed against budgets with built-in standards of achievement (e.g. for patients being transported to a particular clinic, they will be picked up and returned within a specific time of their appointment so that they are not kept waiting at the hospital for hours on end).

GP commissioning: what is it?

GP commissioning is a broad concept and may be regarded as a different way to engage in the planning, monitoring and procurement of care.

Prior to April 2000, all GPs commissioned care for individual patients via the consultation process. Some GPs joined with local colleagues and their health authority to form commissioning groups, whereas others purchased care directly for their patients as fundholders. At its simplest, a group of GPs advised their health authority on the commissioning of local healthcare. The GPs were either local medical committee (LMC) members, who formed small commissioning subcommittees, or a group of neighbouring practices who wished to have a say in how the health authority acted on their behalf.

A major reform of the NHS by the Labour Government on 1 April 1999 was the replacement of GP fundholding with commissioning by a primary care group or primary care trust. This involves general practitioners, other healthcare professionals, community groups and members of the public meeting together to discuss, identify, plan and commission healthcare services to meet the needs of the local community. Any such local plan must meet with the requirements of that area's health improvement programme. Any commissioned healthcare must be of the highest quality, so will be monitored by either the Commission for Health Improvement or the National Institute for Clinical Excellence (NICE) (*see* Chapter 1).

There are similar models of commissioning, although with some differences, in each country of the UK.

Principles of good primary care

There are five principles of good primary healthcare, namely quality, fairness, accountability, responsiveness and efficiency.

Quality

• All those working in primary care should be knowledgeable about the medical conditions they are likely to encounter as a result of their work, and skilled in both treatment and prevention.

• Professionals should be knowledgeable about the communities with whom they are working.

• When working with other NHS or health-related bodies (e.g. social services), those working in primary care should be aware of what is happening outside their own field and work towards delivering a service without gain.

- Premises and facilities should be of a good standard, up to date, well maintained and safe.

Fairness

- Services should be consistent in range and quality across the country.
- Primary care should receive an appropriate share of NHS resources.

Accountability

- Services should be reasonably accessible when clinically needed.
- Necessary services should be available to people regardless of age, sex, ethnicity, disability or health status.

Responsiveness

- Services should reflect the needs and choices of those using them.
- Services should reflect the health and needs of the local population.

Efficiency

- Primary care services should be based on evidence of medical effectiveness.
- Primary care resources should be used effectively.

The New NHS: modern, dependable

Phasing out of fundholding

As part of its 10-year plan for an improved NHS for the twenty-first century, the Government's White Paper announced the end of fundholding and the internal market. While retaining the innovative nature of fundholding, the intention is to make the best features of the scheme available to the *whole* population, and to break down the barriers between services.

Primary care groups

Primary care groups (PCGs) consist of:

- general practitioners
- nurses
- community groups involved in primary care.

Together they have the responsibility for commissioning healthcare services for the local community. A typical PCG will serve a population of approximately 105 000 – 108 000, but the size is flexible and determined by local circumstances. A primary care group is responsible for:

- contributing to the health authority's health improvement programme
- commissioning health services for its population within the health improvement programme parameters
- promoting the health of the local population
- monitoring the services that patients receive
- developing primary care in the local area
- working closely with social services to fully integrate primary and community health services
- ensuring public involvement in primary healthcare decisions.

Primary care groups are managed by a board consisting of:

- a majority of general practitioners (between four and seven)
- community or practice nurses (one or two)
- a representative from the local authority social services department
- one lay member
- one health authority non-executive director.

They also have a chief executive who is appointed by the health authority.

Box 12.1 Data for an average PCG

Patient population	107 000
Number of practices per PCG	19
Practices that were formerly fundholding	47%
Practices formerly involved in joint commissioning	38%
Number of PCGs per health authority	4.8
Approximate expenditure per year:	
Hospital and community health services	£50m
Prescribing	£10m
Practice infrastructure	£2m

Source: Department of Health/Audit Commission Survey, Spring 1999.

Primary care trusts

Primary care groups are now being encouraged to take on the status of a primary care trust (PCT). The NHS Plan indicates that all primary care groups will be expected to become PCTs by 2004. The first wave of PCTs emerged in April 2000. The transition from PCG to PCT involves four levels of responsibility, increasing with each level. Primary care groups are expected to move from Level One to Level Four, and then become independent of the health authority (*see* Chapter 1 for further information).

Links between health and social care

The 1997 *New NHS* reforms proposed a number of important steps to promote more effective links and closer working relationships between health and social services. The NHS Plan is designed to achieve still closer working relationships and integrated care between health and social services, and this has already been achieved in some cases.

Care trusts

The NHS Plan proposes that a different level of primary care trust should be created, which will have the effect of providing even more closely integrated care. The management structure of a PCT will be changed, thus ensuring that both organisations are represented. This new style of NHS trust is known as a 'care trust'.

The patient and the receptionist

From the patient's point of view there are no major changes to services, since they are all still available, but they should now be more efficient as they are delivered according to the Patient's Charter. The Patient's Charter is a document that sets out the standard of service to be provided in layman's language.

Receptionists who are arranging access to services will find that procedures depend on local arrangements (i.e. whether the particular service has gained trust status or whether it is still under the management of the health authority). Set procedures can only be specified by referring to the local offices of the ambulance service, social or community services. It is advisable for staff responsible for arranging transport to visit ambulance headquarters to see at first hand how requests for transport are processed.

As a result of the growth of the primary healthcare sector, the role of the receptionist, clerical and secretarial staff, both in the hospital and in general practice, is becoming increasingly complex as the changes are effected. No longer do staff merely 'go between' the doctor and patient, but they must now liaise with hospital departments, community and social services. Every few months another department or service moves, changes its name, and its personnel change their function or role. It is important for all staff to understand the difficulties experienced in other sectors of health and social care provision as they cope with the fundamental changes that are going on around them.

Although doctors' surgery staff may have been recognised as part of the primary healthcare team for some time, their importance as key members in providing a communication link is growing with the size of the team and the increased variety of necessary points of contact. Similarly, surgery and hospital staff need to be aware of their new role as the Government puts a greater emphasis on health promotion.

The primary healthcare team

The change of emphasis from institutionalised healthcare provision to management by smaller sections within the services generates a greater need for deliberate integration of the various services so that patients are presented with 'seamless' health and social care.

Staff increasingly become involved in dealing with queries, passing messages, and ensuring that the patients released from long-term institutionalised care, or fresh from surgical procedures, receive the service that they need from the various members of the extended primary healthcare team.

From the 1960s, as health authorities built health centres, accommodation was provided for the community, social and other services, including chiropody, dental services and dispensaries. This made it easier for doctors and receptionists to communicate with, for example, community staff, because they were likely to meet in the health centre. In the last few years there has been a general move to 'attach' community staff to specific surgeries where the premises are privately owned by the doctors. A message-book is kept in reception so that messages can be picked up easily, and office space is made available.

The benefits of better communication have been supplemented by developing primary healthcare team meetings. These may have a strong clinical flavour, where doctors and health visitors, midwives and social workers discuss the needs of specific patients. Alternatively, meetings where strategies are developed for defining and maintaining management and administration of the team would also include reception and administration staff. It is essential to have a chairperson to control the agenda so that the subject areas are of interest to everyone. Even if meetings are only held monthly, getting together a group of up to 40 people on a regular basis can be extremely difficult. It is important, therefore, to produce brief minutes so that those who are unable to attend can follow up issues with colleagues.

The primary healthcare team in its broadest sense includes doctors, the practice manager, practice nurses, nurse practitioner, reception, secretarial and other administrative staff, health visitors, midwives, community nursing staff, social workers, community psychiatric nurses and any other nursing specialists. Within this team, however, there are other teams (e.g. receptionists, practice nurses, practice secretaries, etc.). Each team should work together for the common good, so it is important for each team member to appreciate the role, purpose and special skills of its members.

Since October 1997, *all* staff working in primary healthcare, including receptionists, secretaries and practice nurses, are eligible to contribute to the NHS Pension Scheme. This development has meant fewer staff changes in the practice team, and has especially encouraged receptionists and secretaries to feel that their skills and experience are recognised and that their employment offers a worthwhile career structure.

The general medical practitioner

The GP is at the centre of primary healthcare. The doctor's surgery represents the entrance to most of the services provided by the NHS, and the GP's responsibility is to maintain the health of patients and their families by treatment, prevention and health education. GPs give personal and continuing care to their patients, and are in a position to build up a relationship of trust. They attend patients both in their consulting room and in their homes. The GP aims to make initial diagnoses of problems presented, to provide treatment as appropriate, or where necessary to refer patients for further professional treatment.

Registrars (trainees)

If the general medical practice is a training practice, the registrar may be part of the medical team. Registrars are fully qualified doctors undergoing the requisite training and gaining expertise in general medical practice.

The practice manager

The practice manager is the person to whom both secretaries and receptionists in general practice are accountable. He or she has a central role in the day-to-day smooth running of the practice to ensure a quality service to the patients. The practice manager is the leader responsible for building, maintaining and co-ordinating the practice team so that the objectives are achieved and tasks completed satisfactorily. He or she also has responsibility for developing and training individuals and helping them to realise their potential. The practice manager is the person to whom secretaries and receptionists will go to discuss any difficulties and problems they experience in the workplace.

The nurse in primary care

The initiative to increase access to primary care, such as walk-in centres, NHS Direct or minor injuries units, has nurses as the initial point of patient contact. Some practices employ nurses to run specialist clinics (e.g. asthma and diabetes clinics), and patients may be offered a direct consultation with the nurse for certain minor conditions. The nurse's role is certainly expanding as they take on more responsibilities. We already have the nurse practitioner role, and a new post of nurse consultant will further enhance the future role of the nurse in primary care.

Community nursing sisters

These used to be known as district nurses because they worked on a geographical basis looking after the nursing needs of patients in their own homes. They are now more often than not attached to a single practice and work with the patients belonging to that practice, or perhaps the patients of two smaller practices. Practice attachment gives them a chance to work more closely in a team with other staff, but has the disadvantage of spreading their work over a very wide area. Occasionally these nurses work in the treatment room of the practice. They are employed by the community health NHS trust, and are fully trained nurses who have gained experience in hospitals before coming to work in the community. They are involved in traditional nursing duties such as treating people who are ill at home with heart failure, acute chest conditions, terminal illness or, increasingly, after early discharge from hospital. These patients may require wound dressings, attention to bowels, prevention of bed sores and so on, and their relatives at home will gain great support from being taught how to help the patient themselves, or just by knowing that someone will be coming in regularly.

Health visitors

The health visitor is a trained nurse with a post-registration qualification, employed by the community health NHS trust, and working mainly as a member of the primary healthcare team. The training of health visitors is rooted in the promotion of health, and they learn to recognise the effects of psychological, social, economic and environmental factors on health. This enables them to fulfil their role in health education and the prevention of disease.

Although health visitors are concerned with all age groups, they have a special responsibility for the under-fives. New-born babies are visited in their own homes, and parents are advised on matters of child health and development. Emphasis is given to the need for immunisation and the value of attending a child health clinic. They are also concerned with other vulnerable groups such as the elderly, the physically and mentally handicapped, single parents, and families under stress. In addition, they may be involved in the provision of health surveillance programmes and research, in which case an age–sex register or other form of database is particularly helpful.

Practice nurses

These nurses form a rapidly growing group of healthcare workers and represent one way in which health services are changing to meet new challenges. They are usually employed by the practice and do most of their work within the treatment room. They are normally fully trained nurses who have gained experience in hospital and other fields before taking up practice work. Practice nurses are employed in traditional work in the treatment room, such as applying dressings, giving injections, syringing ears and removing sutures. The range of their activity is changing to include helping to run health promotion clinics, and assisting with child health surveillance and minor surgery. They are thus often specially trained in the management of chronic illness such as asthma, diabetes and hypertension. Practice nurses are beginning to use some of the tools that were traditionally used only by the doctor, such as ophthalmoscopes, stethoscopes, auriscopes and vaginal speculae. Further important extensions of their work include counselling, listening and reassuring.

Nurse practitioners

Nurse practitioners are nurses with specialist training which allows them to practise independently. In some cases they take on responsibilities similar to those of junior medical staff, and in general practice they may run clinics and assess priorities.

Midwives

Midwives have a central role in the care of pregnant women. They are fully trained nurses who have subsequently completed a prolonged midwifery course. They are employed by the community health NHS trust and they form part of the team with hospital obstetricians, general practitioners and health visitors concerned with antenatal care, antenatal preparation, intrapartum care, delivery, and postpartum care of the mother and infant. They sometimes run antenatal clinics with doctors, and conduct normal deliveries in hospital and occasionally in the home. They are also very much involved in the postpartum care of mothers who are discharged home early after delivery.

Social workers

In about one in five consultations a doctor becomes involved in discussions and advice about personal relationships, work, social benefits, social support or other financial matters. These are important features of primary care, but just as the doctor will want to call upon the special skills of nurses for some problems, so he will want to use a social worker's skills for the issues listed above.

For example, if a young single mother is taken ill, the problem extends beyond the immediate care of a sick woman and involves a healthy child as well. If an elderly person living alone has a minor stroke which limits their independence by making it difficult to cook, clean or shop, another type of problem arises that might best be solved by a home help, meals on wheels or laundry services. The social worker will help to assess the need for this service, and to set up these forms of care if they are needed. Again, if family tensions put the wife or children at risk, supervision and counselling may be required, and the problem is most likely to be dealt with by a social worker.

There are some specialised social workers. These include psychiatric social workers, who have an important role in the involuntary admission of the psychiatrically ill and in helping and supporting the long-term sick, such as patients who are schizophrenics, or those with senile dementia who live in the community.

Community psychiatric nurses

Community psychiatric nurses belong to a profession which, although still in its infancy, is of increasing importance. Their role has developed with the trend towards rehabilitating and caring for the mentally infirm in the community. Although they may be used in psychiatric hospitals, they are largely involved in providing support and treatment in collaboration with general practitioners. They tend to act as independant clinical practitioners themselves, backed by both consultants and general practitioners, with the object of restricting long-term hospital treatment to only the severest cases.

Pharmacists

We saw in another section how doctors and pharmacists relate to each other in terms of their activities with prescriptions. Many patients go first to the pharmacist with their complaint, and may never need to see the doctor. Others are advised by the pharmacist that a consultation is necessary. Communication between the two professions is very important.

Optometrists

These are specialist health professionals who test eyes and prescribe lenses to correct sight problems. They are more commonly referred to as 'opticians'. A 'dispensing optician' fits and sells glasses but does not test eyes. An ophthalmic optician specialises in making glasses, testing eyes and prescribing appropriate lenses.

Home helps

Home helps play a vital role in enabling the elderly to stay in their homes for as long as possible. Their role is to perform those domestic tasks – such as shopping, washing, cleaning and collecting pensions – which the elderly can no longer undertake because of infirmity. They have no clinical responsibility, but their visits provide a friendly and caring link with the outside world. It is usually the social services department of the local authority that organises their work.

Home care teams

We have seen that some teams consist of people employed by the practice, whilst others consist of people employed by the health authorities. There is yet another arm of support, namely voluntary organisations. A particularly good example of this is the hospice which provides care for the terminally ill. Doctors and nurses working in this field, supported mainly by charity, develop a particular expertise and have teams that can visit patients in their own homes by arrangement with the general practitioner.

Other members of the healthcare team

Physiotherapists diagnose and treat patients' difficulties with movement, especially with regard to joints, and assist with rehabilitation after injury. Until recently they worked mainly in hospitals, but an increasing number now work in the community. GPs have direct access to their services.

Social workers can help many patients with problems in non-medical areas of their lives (e.g. living conditions, debts or problems with relationships or child care). The intervention of social workers at an early stage can often help in tackling patients' problems, although these may be closely related to medical conditions for which they consult their doctor. In some areas, GPs employ their own social worker because of the support he or she can give to patients who visit their doctor because they do not know where else to go.

Counsellors may be employed by GPs or attend their surgeries for designated sessions. Early intervention by a counsellor who has time to listen to patients' non-medical problems can help to avert a critical situation.

Dietitians and other care staff advise on the best diet for particular medical conditions. Some health centres and GP practices have a dietitian who attends for designated sessions, working closely with members of the primary healthcare team.

Occupational therapists help patients to resume a normal life after mental or physical illness, through activity-based treatments and the provision of aids to living. They will also assess what alterations are needed to enable elderly or disabled people to continue living at home.

Speech and language therapists help patients who have communication difficulties, especially after stroke or injury. They are trained to diagnose and treat all forms of speech disabilities and disorders of language and articulation in children.

Chiropodists play an important part in helping the elderly (who frequently have debilitating toe and foot problems) to maintain an active role in the community.

Audiometricians do much to help those with hearing disabilities to live a normal and active life.

There is a large variety of other skilled workers who, from time to time, become part of the team. Experts such as chiropodists, dietitians, physiotherapists, clinical psychologists, pharmacists, and so on, may be involved.

The principal skill of clinical psychologists is in the realm of personal development and interpersonal relationships. They can help with behavioural problems in children and teenagers, helping people to cope with life's difficulties, marital problems, and so on.

Other specialist nurses

Specialist nurses working in the community also include the following:

- school nurse
- stoma care nurse
- paediatric nurse
- geriatric nurse
- local authority clinic nurse.

The Terms of Service for family health services practitioners

General practitioners working in the NHS have a contract with the health authority or health board/health and social services board to provide general medical services for their NHS patients. Receptionists and secretaries should have an understanding of the main Terms of Service which may concern their daily work. The Terms of Service for doctors in general practice require a GP principal to:

*   provide medical care to anyone whom he or she has accepted as a patient

*   be available to his or her patients at all times or arrange a competent doctor to provide care in his or her absence

*   be available at the surgery or visit patients at times agreed with the health authority. A full-time principal is expected to work at least 26 hours each week (this does not include on-call hours)

*   offer in writing to patients aged 75 years and over an annual consultation and a domiciliary visit, to assess whether any treatment is required

*   provide a consultation within 28 days of registration for all newly registered patients

*   provide premises adequate for the delivery of medical care

*   employ staff who are suitably qualified and competent to undertake the duties required of them

*   ensure that practice staff receive continuing training

*   provide a practice information leaflet for patients

*   send an annual report to the health authority giving details of the staff, premises, use of hospital services and prescribing arrangements

*   have in place and operate a practice-based complaints procedure

*   have a written Practice Charter.

In 1995, the Department of Health agreed changes to the terms and conditions of the contract which made it easier for GPs not to see patients out of hours. GPs are now able to opt out of organising and providing 24-hour care altogether, as long as another GP has been identified who will provide that service to their patients. In the past GPs were paid a higher fee if they covered their own patients out of hours and if they visited them in their own home rather than asking them to come to the surgery. However, there is now a single fee for night visits, and GPs are paid the same rate for seeing any patient, whether or not they are on their list, and whether they are seeing them at home or at the surgery.

Co-operatives

Many GPs are forming rotas to share on-call work. The GP co-operatives usually involve more than 10 GPs and generally vary in size from 15 GPs to more than 200, covering areas from small towns to a hundred miles or so.

Deputising services

Some practices are making greater use of deputising services, which are run by private companies, whereby GPs pay the service a fee and the deputising service arranges for another GP to cover their patients out of hours.

Emergency centres

Many co-operatives and deputising services have set up emergency centres to which patients have to travel, or which they are able to telephone for advice. These centres may be based at a local practice, in a local hospital or in purpose-built premises. They cover a number of practices, and are staffed by GPs and occasionally also by practice nurses.

Health promotion

Approximately 20 years ago, health education was a new field seeking to make information about health matters available to anyone who wanted it. Health education councils generated literature and visited surgeries, schools and hospitals to circulate information. In the last five years there has been an increase in health promotion in doctors' surgeries which has supplemented health education. Every opportunity is taken to draw attention to health issues, advise individuals to bring them to a point of decision about making changes in their lifestyle, and then give out literature to educate further on how and why to make such changes.

Health promotion draws attention to the need to change, and educates sufficiently to enable a patient to make an informed choice to change. Support during the change process and further education with literature must then follow. The terms 'education' and 'promotion' refer to different aspects, but to effect change in patient behaviour the two must work hand in hand.

General practitioners and healthcare providers have been required to extend their services into promotion of health, as well as looking after the sick. Surgeries have implemented health promotion clinics, such as well-man and well-woman clinics, where patients are asked for details of their lifestyle and given advice on how they might prevent ill health by changes to their diet, drinking habits, smoking habits, exercise levels and so on. Where needs such as help in giving up smoking are identified, specific clinics are then provided in some surgeries, so that patients benefit from peer group support.

However, all members of the primary healthcare team, including receptionists and secretaries, are now required to be far more aware of promoting health. Just as one would find it difficult to accept advice from an obviously overweight practice nurse advising that one must lose at least two stones in weight in the next six months, it is important that healthcare staff present a healthy image – which may include not being seen smoking – to back up the message that the practitioners and other health professionals give out daily.

Patient waiting-areas should be used to the full to promote health, with good-quality notices tidily displayed on notice-boards, and to educate by leaflets that are available for patients to read while they are waiting, or to take home with them. It may be the practice nurse's responsibility to maintain notice-boards and supplies of leaflets, but it is important that receptionists keep their eyes open and draw the nurse's attention to notice-boards that are looking unkempt or leaflet supplies that are running low.

General practices have also found that 'open days' are an excellent opportunity to give out health promotion messages, when patients are invited into the surgery, perhaps on a Saturday afternoon, to have blood pressure and cholesterol checks, and so on.

The educational aspect is supported by most schools, which ask health visitors and social workers to speak to children and answer questions about what they can do to help themselves. Schools may also invite specific organisations, such as ASH (anti-smoking) or local AIDS charities to educate students about their particular area of expertise.

Since there are 1001 sources of educational information, the role of staff is to be aware of where materials can be obtained for a wide range of subjects, so that literature can be accessed without undue delay. Where literature is not available free of charge, details of costs might be kept on record together with the addresses and contact numbers.

The Government is making funding available for health promotion in surgeries by paying doctors who achieve targets for health promotion, but it is very difficult to audit the results. The range of effects on individual lives that might contribute to ill health makes it impossible to generalise about how effective any one particular message might have been. However, research to date shows that eating 'healthily', taking regular exercise and practising moderation in alcohol intake, together with refraining from smoking, all contribute to remaining healthier for longer. Where large-scale health promotion in partnership with health education has been government sponsored, as in Finland, treatment for and deaths from heart disease have been reduced.

Therefore it is part of the role of the receptionist to support initiatives to promote better health, not only by being aware of the advice given out by doctors and health professionals, but also by advising patients to attend health promotion clinics or events put on by the surgery, and by themselves presenting a healthy image to patients.

Local authority social services

Major local authorities have a social services committee, with an appointed director in charge of its social services department, who co-ordinates and administers the authority's social services.

Secretaries and receptionists will inevitably be asked by patients for information and advice about social services provision, and should have the relevant information readily available to enable them to deal with such queries in a helpful, positive way.

Structure and social services provided

Figure 12.1 shows the structure of a typical social services department. The organisation of the department will vary from one area to another, but there are usually at least five main sections of a social services department:

- residential services
- fieldwork services
- provision of training facilities
- hospital social work
- administration.

The following is a summary of the services provided by social services committees:

- *care of the elderly* – this includes both fieldwork services carried out within the community and residential care

- *care of the physically handicapped* – this includes blind, deaf, dumb, hearing difficulties, spastic, epileptic, paraplegics and other disabled people

- *social work advice to the homeless* – this includes provision of permanent accommodation, care of homeless families, advice and help on prevention of homelessness, and bed-and-breakfast accommodation.

Note: Those who are homeless are 'priority'. 'Priority' means anyone who has one or more children living with them, anyone who is made homeless (e.g. by fire or flood), any household which includes one or more people who are elderly or mentally/physically handicapped, or suffer from physical disability, battered wives, and pregnant women. The homeless are also divided into those made *homeless by chance* and those made *homeless intentionally*.

- *Child care services* – child care protection/supervision; acceptance of parental responsibility for children committed into care of the local authority; control of residential units; admission units; reception centres; residential nurseries; children's homes; community homes with education on the premises and classifying homes; adoption services; child abuse/prevention of child abuse services.

- *Social work and family casework dealing with mental disorder* – provision of social workers; adult training centres; workshops; residential accommodation (hostels).

- *Day care for children under five years of age* – provision of day nurseries, supervision of private nurseries and childminders.

- *Provision of home carers*.

- *Care of unsupported mothers* – including residential care.

- *Hospital social workers* – provision of social work services for hospital patients.

- *Work in the field of alcohol and drug abuse*.

It will have been noted that social services offer a wide range of services for people who are at risk or who have a high level of need, and aim to protect and support vulnerable people by helping them to live independently.

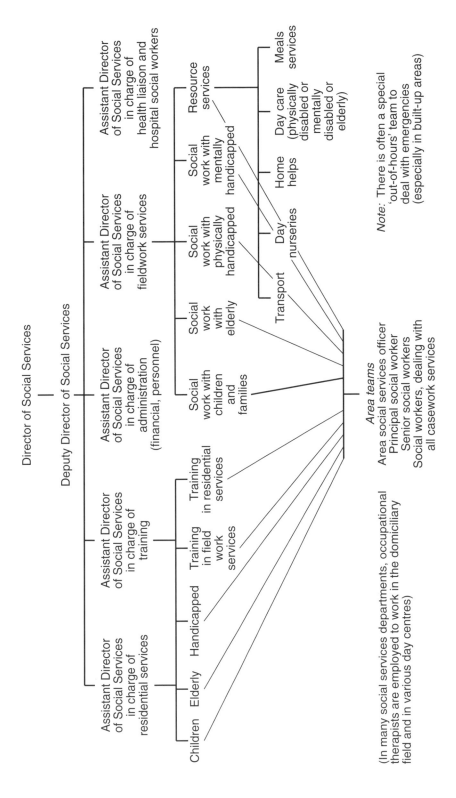

Figure 12.1 The structure of a typical social services department.

Assessment

An assessment of needs is conducted by a member of specialist staff in the home, in hospital, or in the social services office. The assessment gives the person concerned the opportunity to discuss their needs.

Social work teams

A team of area social workers undertakes all of the casework for family and clients, so that problems can be considered as a whole, thus leading to family social services, helping all kinds of social problems in the family. Teams are composed of specialist social workers (e.g. specialists in child care, mental illness or handicap, physical handicap, and care of the elderly). It is the area social work team which usually co-ordinates the allocation of the following:

- home carers
- meals on wheels
- day-nursery places
- vacancies in residential homes for the elderly
- residential accommodation for children.

Health and social services liaison

Social services work in close liaison with the local health authority to provide support and help in the community to patients recently discharged from hospital, or suffering from a disabling condition. The necessary adaptations, gadgets and aids for these people that are vital for their rehabilitation are supplied by the occupational therapy section of the social services department.

A community physician who is a specialist in community medicine is responsible for liaison between health and social services. Social workers now visit medical practices and health centres, where they meet general practitioners, health visitors, community nurses and school nurses working from these centres.

Community care

Social services departments will continue to work closely with health authorities to plan and provide 'care packages' to give the support that people need to help in their daily lives, and may be available from local government and health authorities. It involves both social and healthcare, and the Government will continue to encourage purchasers and providers to work with local authority partners to ensure that arrangements for community care work effectively. One of the major aims of community care is to enable people to maximise their independence by living in their own home for as long as possible, and when this is no longer practicable, to find them a home-like place to live.

Community care trusts

Community care trusts work in partnership with GPs and others to provide well-run services. Teams of highly skilled staff work in many different places, including patients' homes, health centres, clinics, GP surgeries, schools and residential and nursing homes. They are able to diagnose and treat both chronic and acute illnesses, and provide rehabilitation and care for those who are dying.

Services include the following:

- district nursing
- health visiting
- school nursing
- child health clinics
- chiropody
- dental care
- rehabilitation and therapy service
- health promotion
- family planning
- well-woman/man services
- loan of equipment for care at home
- children's medical services and development assessment
- health services for children with special needs.

Many trusts also provide a hospital-at-home scheme for children and older people, which may enable patients to be discharged home sooner, or perhaps avoid hospitalisation altogether.

Patients are usually referred by their GP or other healthcare staff.

Mental health services

Local authorities provide a wide range of services, including community care services, for people who require mental health services. Local community care charters give information about the services and standards expected from local social services departments, which help to ensure higher standards of social care for people with mental illness.

Local authorities should have a charter covering community services for people with mental health problems which are responsive to local needs. Patients and carers have a right to know what community care services are available and the standards of performance that they can expect to receive. Community care charters should cover information about the following:

- assessments and care management

- performance standards for services

- how to complain

- how local authorities monitor performance.

Many NHS trusts provide specialist mental health services for people who are experiencing mental health problems. In addition, they may provide specialist services for people who have learning disabilities and need special care and support to develop life skills.

The trusts provide a number of specialised services, including the following:

- inpatient and outpatient psychiatry

- psychotherapy

- psychology

- vocational employment services

- specialist addiction and eating disorder services.

Services for people with mental health problems are provided by highly skilled staff, and range from community mental health teams, and day care to secure inpatient wards.

Care Programme Approach

The Care Programme Approach is the way in which specialist mental health services are delivered to those who need them, and patients can expect the following:

- an assessment of their health and social care needs

- a written plan to meet those needs

- to be involved in drawing up their care plan

- a regular review of their care plan

- to have a named mental health worker (a care co-ordinator or key-worker) who is responsible for the patient's care under the Care Programme Approach.

New rights for carers

From 1 April 1996, carers were given new rights under a new law called the Carers Recognition and Services Act (otherwise known as the Carers Act). This Act entitles carers to an assessment in their own right. Social services departments will have to listen to carers, record their views and take into account the result of the carer's assessment when they decide what services to bring to the person who is being cared for. The Carers Act states that carers are people who look after and support sick, elderly and disabled relatives and friends, providing a substantial amount of care on a regular basis.

Summary

The foregoing account is intended to stress the importance to secretaries and receptionists of having sources of information at their fingertips so that they are able to answer, with knowledge and understanding, the numerous and diverse questions that will be put to them by patients and their relatives.

   At the time of writing, many changes are taking place in both primary care and social care of patients. As a result, staff should ensure that they have an understanding of the changes taking place so that they are able to answer all of the queries that may be put to them.

13

Audit, health economics and ensuring quality for the medical receptionist and secretary

Introduction

Receptionists and secretaries working in the healthcare field will no doubt be aware of the emergence of new concepts and buzzwords or phrases for a wide variety of initiatives and processes, all aimed at benefiting the patient. The most important of these issues is considered to give the reader an underpinning knowledge and understanding of concepts that are influencing the NHS today.

Audit

Receptionists and secretaries in their day-to-day activities can consider what they do and if they can do it better to provide a quality service to patients. This may include the following:

1 identifying or defining criteria and standards in order to answer the question 'What are we doing/trying to achieve for our patients?'
2 collecting data on current performance (i.e. the care and/or service given and its effects on patients). Are patients satisfied?

Figure 13.1

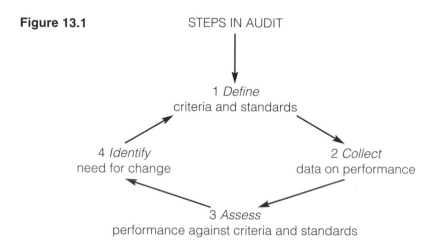

3   assessing performance against criteria to determine whether standards have been met and objectives achieved
4   identifying the need for change or improvement in patient care.

The importance of audit

Decision making can only be truly effective when it is based on accurate record keeping and information about various activities. For example, receptionists may be asked to keep records of the numbers of patients seen at the surgery or in the hospital clinic. This is important in decision making to improve the quality of care or service to patients:

- to introduce a new clinic

- to extend the length of the surgery or clinic

- to check that the current consultation system is working satisfactorily in the best interests of both doctors and patients

- to increase staffing levels.

Secretaries and receptionists may feel that the information or statistics which are kept to help decision making are never-ending, but it must be remembered that the conclusions drawn may affect all members of the team and foster a feeling of team spirit and involvement. This in turn will create a professional and caring team that plays an important part in the delivery of a high standard of service and healthcare.

Health economics and cost-effective medicine

Although it is appreciated that readers of this book are unlikely to become involved in these processes, an insight will provide an understanding of some of the dominant political and economic issues facing the NHS and healthcare today. The UK, like many other nations, has experienced a rapid increase in healthcare expenditure, and with it health economics.

Health economics

Economics is concerned with the way in which people earn their living and how they spend their earnings, particularly on goods and services. Health economics is defined as the way in which resources are allocated to health-related issues and the increasing cost of providing a quality healthcare system. As expenditure on healthcare has increased dramatically over the past 30 years, it is not surprising that health economics has emerged as a speciality in its own right and has shown a rapid expansion.

Economics can be divided into two main areas:

- macroeconomics
- microeconomics.

Macroeconomics is concerned with the functioning of the whole economy. Microeconomics is concerned with the functioning of individual parts of the economic system (e.g. the price of a particular product or service, or the behaviour of an individual organisation/institution, and so on). Healthcare is part of the microeconomic system concerned with the effects of expenditure in supplying the needs and demands made upon it. It focuses the choices made by individuals within the health system.

Evidence-based and cost-effective medicine

The philosophy of evidence-based medicine encourages the medical profession to base the practice of medicine on proven effective treatments or services which are of benefit to, and in the best interests of, patients, yet which at the same time consider the cost-effectiveness of such treatment. It is based on evidence resulting from medical research, comparisons and outcomes of clinical audit. Consideration is given to the cost of providing such treatment, the availability of funds and the quality of patient care.

Private Finance Initiative

The Private Finance Initiative (PFI), which was first announced in the 1992 Budget, is intended to harness private-sector management expertise and efficiency in delivering public services. In the NHS it has included the building and servicing of new district general hospital facilities as well as a range of smaller projects.

For example, some trusts have been able to replace ageing X-ray equipment through a PFI contract, and as a result now have state-of-the-art scanning equipment in their imaging department. It has been suggested that private contractors may play a key role in the new generation of 'fast-track' treatment centres through PFI style contracts.

The Department of Health has standardised contracts with PFI consortia – specially created companies which negotiate contracts on behalf of building and finance managers.

The scheme enables the NHS to harness private-sector expertise, allowing NHS management to concentrate on delivering cost-effective clinical services and ultimately providing better value for money.

Plans to redevelop existing hospitals by providing updated facilities and more sophisticated diagnostic equipment are going ahead, with finance being made available through the public–private partnership (PPP) initiative.

Clinical governance

Clinical governance is a statutory duty aimed at 'ensuring that all NHS organisations have in place proper processes for continuously monitoring and improving clinical audit'. Clinicians and managers will be expected to understand their individual and collective responsibilities for assuring accountability for the quality of patient healthcare, and take on a legal responsibility for standards of health service treatment.

One tool of clinical governance designed to improve the quality of medical care might be clinical audit, which evaluates the results and effectiveness of treatment. In this way it is possible to identify improvements, or the need for them, which have occurred in medical practice over a period of time, and to identify medical standards and guidelines based on research evidence. Clinical governance means that every healthcare professional should be responsible and accountable for his or her own personal standards of practice.

National Institute for Clinical Excellence (NICE)

NICE was set up in April 1999 as a new body that aims to promote the highest quality of treatment and technology in the NHS, and the cost-effectiveness of NHS services. It gives guidelines on best clinical practice in the NHS to those commissioning NHS services including:

- health authorities
- primary care groups
- primary care trusts
- patients and their carers.

NICE is a partnership between the Department of Health, the NHS, health professionals and patients. Guidelines set by NICE will be used countrywide and will help to end the geographical variations in care that have developed in recent years.

National Clinical Assessment Authority (NCAA)

This is a new national body that will operate from April 2001. It will provide a central point of contact for the NHS when concerns about a doctor's performance are raised. The authority will give advice to NHS hospitals, health authorities and trusts to make sure that the performance of doctors is checked, and action will be taken to ensure that doctors are practising safely, thus ensuring the quality of medical practice.

National Service Frameworks (NSF)

This is another new initiative designed to help to establish clear national standards to improve quality and reduce unacceptable variations in the standards of care and treatment. The NSF for coronary heart disease and mental health and the NHS Cancer Plan and an NSF for diabetes will be published later in 2001.

Frameworks are founded on knowledge-based practice and are designed to promote partnership working between:

- those who use and those who provide the service

- different clinicians and practitioners

- different parts of the NHS

- the NHS and local government.

Summary

Many initiatives designed to ensure the accountability and quality of patient care and efficient medical practice have been introduced in recent years. A statutory body developed by the Government came into being at the end of 1999 to support and promote quality standards, and to keep a watchful eye on NHS service activity. This was the Commission for Health Improvement (CHI).

The main role of the CHI is to concentrate on clinical quality issues, and it will ensure that other quality mechanisms for improving the quality of service are proving to be efficient and effective. It will also ensure that variations in standards throughout the NHS are minimised.

Conclusion

Although they are not directly involved in the concepts discussed in this chapter, receptionists and secretaries form an integral part of a healthcare team which is committed to providing patients with high-quality and cost-effective care. It is important to remember that every member of the team is involved in collecting the data necessary to assess the quality of care, and if change is indicated as an outcome of audit, then teamwork is essential to achieving the wider context of quality in healthcare provision.

14

Training and development

Training and development should also be considered as ways of improving your personal effectiveness. Before we consider this in more detail, it is important to distinguish between the following:

- training
- education
- development.

Training is a systematic process for developing the skills, knowledge and attitudes applied to a specific type of work. It is the process of bringing a person to an agreed standard of competence by practice or instruction.

Education is the process of acquiring background knowledge and skills. It does not have to be specific to a particular area of work.

Development is a course of action which enables individuals to realise their potential for growth and promotion in an organisation.

Well-trained receptionists and secretaries are valued members of the work team, and are better able to understand, appreciate and contribute to the smooth running of the medical practice or hospital department.

Excellent training courses are available, and may be provided as in-house training in the work environment, or by external training providers (e.g. health authorities and colleges of further education) (*see* Appendix 3). Training courses leading to a recognised qualification may necessitate attendance at a college on a day release basis, or may be provided as short training courses which take place in the evening.

Why train?

The reasons for training staff are varied, but generally they will fall into one of the following categories:

1   induction needs of new staff:

  • introduction to the practice, the practice team and practice objectives

  • information about the workplace and conditions of employment

  • initial job training

2   to help staff to improve their performance at work:

  • where staff need further training to enable them to do their job at the required level of competence

3   further job training:

  • to give fuller job-related training in specific areas/tasks

4   personal development:

  • training provided where staff wish to develop their career (e.g. by attending a course to gain a professional qualification)

5   retraining:

  • where the nature of the job changes and retraining is necessary to enable the individual to carry out the new work competently

6   policy implementation:

  • staff training may be necessary to ensure that national criteria are implemented

7   response to organisational change:

  • training is necessary where staff are required to respond to changes that affect their jobs (e.g. introduction of new technology, improving teamwork, teambuilding, etc.).

Training strategies

There are six main training strategies that are appropriate to the needs of receptionists and secretaries:

  •   *on-the-job*: may be carried out by the individual's immediate supervisor in the workplace

- *planned organisational experience*: in-house training, such as a special project to investigate a problem (e.g. appointments system not working well) and make recommendations for improvement

- *in-house courses*: suitable for short-term training needs to target a specific area, and carried out by the individual's immediate supervisor or an external trainer

- *off-the-job (external courses)*: regular attendance at a college or training centre offering specific courses/qualifications

- *open/distance learning*: training courses designed to give greater flexibility and suitable where regular attendance is impractical

- *on-line learning*: more and more educational providers are not only providing traditional tutorial support for open and distance learning training courses, but are also offering on-line and web-based support as well as opportunities to join in discussions with tutors and other students.

Self-development

Self-development is the development of yourself, by yourself, through a deliberate process of learning from experience. This definition assumes that you need to organise it for yourself, rather than expect other people to be responsible for your development. If you do not take responsibility for your own development, who else will? The door to development is locked – you are the keyholder!

Your manager is responsible for providing you with development opportunities, but it is always up to the individual to take the opportunities on offer and make something of them.

The NHS Plan

The NHS Plan confirms the need for employers to provide training opportunities for individual members of staff to further their careers. The deadline of April 2001 was stated for employers to organise a training and development plan for all of their staff which should be linked to appraisal systems.

The NHS Plan has promised an individual leaning account (ILA) for all staff who do not have a professional qualification, or training, to NVQ Level Two or Three. Both NVQs and ILA offer a means of assuring quality standards in the workplace. ILAs have been developed by the Department of Education and Employment and provide the opportunity for learning about many aspects of healthcare.

NHS staff are able to apply for a place on this scheme.

National Vocational Qualifications (NVQs)

National Vocational Qualifications (NVQs) were introduced in order to replace the varied range of occupational qualifications with an assessed set of standards, which are created by national training and employer-led organisations. These organisations represent an occupational or industrial sector.

NVQs provide a flexible means of obtaining a qualification. There is virtually no time limit, and there are no examinations. They are composed of units which describe the skills and knowledge which are necessary to carry out a job efficiently, and they may be described as a statement of performance.

More and more training and development programmes and learning materials are designed to provide the underpinning knowledge and understanding which facilitate the achievement of competence towards NVQs (SNVQs in Scotland).

NVQs (and SNVQs) are based on what people need to be able to do in order to carry out their jobs competently. They are work-based competences, which are assessed in the workplace. The qualifications are based on completion of units and elements and achievement of stated standards of performance criteria.

NVQs (and SNVQs) are assessed on the production of evidence of achievement, and secretaries and receptionists who wish to achieve NVQs (or SNVQs) should gather evidence in the form of a 'portfolio'. A portfolio is a collection of evidence demonstrating competence which can be based on previous as well as current learning.

The system is accredited by the Qualifications Curriculum Authority (QCA), which was set up in 1997 to regulate all external qualifications in England, Wales, Northern Ireland and Scotland.

All awarding bodies (e.g. the RSA Examinations Board) that wish to accredit national qualifications must apply to the QCA to achieve nationally accredited awarding body status.

NHS staff without a professional qualification are eligible to apply for a place on this scheme. All such staff will have access to an ILA of £150 or dedicated training to NVQ (level 2 or 3). As a result of this investment, it is anticipated that the NHS will better use its staff, including healthcare assistants, pharmacy technicians, operating department practitioners and administrative staff, thus providing an improved standard of patient care.

A national framework is in place to implement this scheme, helping employers to make work-related training available to their staff.

Career structure

Secretaries and receptionists working in the field of healthcare are in a position, with their experience and further training, to progress to achieve the position of senior secretary or receptionist, and could well be considered to be sufficiently competent to progress further to a supervisory or management role within the organisation.

An opportunity to discuss career development and any training needs could be identified at your annual performance appraisal, and a personal development plan arranged.

Summary

Training and development contribute to developing your personal effectiveness as a medical secretary or receptionist, and also to being a more effective and highly valued member of the work team.

There are several professional organisations and associations that offer recognised qualifications. Your practice manager, training manager or your local college will be able to provide you with further information.

15

Complementary medicine

Introduction

This chapter on *complementary* (or *alternative*) *medicine* is included because the term is recognised by the public and acknowledged by the medical profession. A term that was used in a published report by the British Medical Association in 1993 was 'non-conventional therapy'. However, this form of treatment is now offered as an alternative or complementary treatment to conventional (orthodox) medicine, and in some instances it is provided under the NHS.

Medical receptionists and secretaries working either for the NHS or in private practice or hospital may be involved in dealing with patients' enquiries about such provision, with the prior approval of the healthcare professionals involved, of course. This chapter aims to give the reader an outline of non-conventional therapies (*see* Appendix 13 for a list of useful addresses), and to provide an overview of some which are practised in the UK.

Acupuncture

This traditional 4000-year-old Chinese healing system came to Europe in the nineteenth century.

Medical or Western acupuncture is based on traditional Chinese medicine, and is practised by doctors on the medical register. It is a 'touch' technique based on the theory of body meridian lines, or lines of force. Needles are inserted along the meridians in order to balance the body's *yin* and *yang* forces and thereby restore or promote the healing forces of the body. Medical or Western acupuncture is also used to achieve anaesthesia. Doctors, physiotherapists and nurses must successfully undertake a two-year course of postgraduate study in order to be registered to practise acupuncture.

Alexander technique

The *Alexander technique* was founded by an Australian actor whose breathing problems affected his career. It is a method of postural correction and re-education in which people are taught to stand and move efficiently.

The *Society of Teachers of the Alexander Technique* supervises training and maintains a code of ethics and a register of teachers.

Aromatherapy

Aromatherapy originated in the Middle East and was introduced to Europe by the Romans. It is a touch technique based on the healing properties of essential plant oils. Holistic aromatherapy uses massage and essential oils to treat emotional and physical problems. Aromatherapy is not a regulated therapy, and individuals may set up as practitioners. However, an Aromatherapy Council was set up in 1991 with the aim of setting standards with 50 hours of clinical training followed by an examination. Success in the latter would give entry to the Register of Qualified Aromatherapists.

Chiropractic

Chiropractic was developed by a Canadian osteopath to treat musculo-skeletal disorders and their effect on the nervous system by manipulation and soft tissue massage. Therapists use spinal X-rays for the diagnosis of mechanical problems. Appropriate exercises and postural advice are given. Qualification is by a five-year full-time degree course followed by one year in a British Chiropractic Association clinic, after which an honorary doctorate of chiropractic is obtained.

Homeopathy

Homeopathy is yet another ancient treatment dating back to the fourth century BC, when Hippocrates suggested that treatment with something that mimics illness might cure it. Patients in Europe have been treated by this principle since the late eighteenth century, and homeopathy is now well established in the UK, with hundreds of medically qualified doctors registered as homeopaths.

Treatment consists of the administration of greatly diluted forms of natural substances that in a healthy person would produce symptoms similar to those which the medicine is prescribed to treat.

The Statutory Faculty of Homeopathy trains and registers medical practitioners in homeopathy.

Hydrotherapy

Although hydrotherapy cannot be referred to as *complementary* medicine, as it is an orthodox treatment practised by appropriately qualified chartered physiotherapists, it is becoming increasingly recognised as an effective therapy. Hydrotherapy consists of physiotherapy exercises and treatment in a warm, shallow pool heated to approximately 35°C. The warmth of the water and the natural buoyancy supporting the limbs enable movements to be carried out which could not normally be performed on dry land.

Hydrotherapy also improves the circulation, relieves pain and stiffness, and improves mobility and posture. It is used mainly in the effective treatment of many locomotor disorders, including rheumatic and arthritic conditions, in addition to pre- and postoperative rehabilitation of joint replacement, spinal surgery, fractures and sports injuries. Hydrotherapy is practised by a registered physiotherapist who has undertaken a post-graduate course in hydrotherapy.

Hypnotherapy

This therapy was first used by the Greeks to treat problems such as anxiety and hysteria. An eighteenth-century Austrian physician, Franz Mesmer, successfully treated people by putting them into a trance. Subsequently, a French physician, Ambrose Lebeaut, developed the technique of hypnosis.

In hypnotherapy, the patient is made to relax with the use of hypnosis. The therapy is aimed at reducing pain, bringing about changes in mental state and making suggestions for relieving symptoms.

Many doctors, dentists and psychologists are clinically trained in hypnotherapy, but anyone can set up as a hypnotherapist, as there is no regulatory body. The duration of training may vary from one or two days to several months. The National School of Hypnotherapy and Psychotherapy offers training courses.

Osteopathy

Osteopathy was founded in the nineteenth century by an American who was both a doctor and an engineer, and the technique arrived in the UK at the beginning of the twentieth century. The first school of osteopathy was established in 1917 in London.

Osteopathy is a system of diagnosis and healing that aims to improve the functioning of the body through its structure. It works primarily through articulation and mobilisation of the musculoskeletal system (the bones and soft tissues of the body) in order to influence the nerve supply, the blood supply, the fluid systems and the energy systems of the body and maximise the body's self-healing ability. Although generally associated with the treatment of back pain and bone disorders, osteopathy is now used to relieve a wide variety of ailments, including digestive, respiratory and circulatory problems, neck pain, joint pain and mobility problems.

Practitioners use mainly gentle manual manipulative methods to restore and maintain biomechanical function.

Osteopathy was the first complementary therapy to be statutorily regulated. The Osteopaths Act of 1993 protects patients from untrained practitioners. Since 1999, all osteopaths have had to be registered with the General Osteopathic Council which holds a list of professional requirements, recognised qualifications and compulsory preregistration training.

Reflexology

Over 5000 years ago, hand and foot massage was practised in China and India. In the nineteenth century an American surgeon noticed that when pressure was applied to certain areas of the hand and foot, partial anaesthesia to the nose and throat was produced, allowing minor surgery to be performed. This concept was developed and introduced to the UK. Reflexology consists of compression and massage techniques using reflex areas of the feet and hands, and is designed to stimulate the blood supply and nerves, thus relieving tension. It may also be used as an indicator of possible problems in various parts of the body.

The Association of Reflexologists gives accreditation to courses in the UK, and the British Reflexology Association is a representative professional organisation. Both organisations have codes of practice and ethics, as well as holding lists of accredited therapists.

Summary

An overview of the most widely used forms of complementary medicine has been given, although it is appreciated that other non-conventional therapies have been found to have a beneficial effect. These include the following:

- herbalism
- massage (touch)
- tai chi (oriental, self-help, postural)
- yoga (oriental, self-help, postural).

Further reading and reference books

Medical secretaries and receptionists should know the sources from which information can be obtained. The following list will be of value.

Medical reference

- *Medical Dictionary – Dorland's Pocket Medical Dictionary*
  Pocket Medical Dictionary, Churchill Livingstone.

- *The Medical Directory* – consists of two volumes containing a directory of all qualified medical practitioners, with addresses, qualifications and posts held. Information about hospitals is also included. There will usually be a recent copy at your place of employment.

- *First Aid Manual* – the authorised manual of St John's Ambulance Association, St Andrew's Ambulance Association and the British Red Cross Society.

- *British National Formulary* – this contains accurate information about all proprietary drugs.

- *MIMS* – a monthly publication listing all proprietary drugs and their uses.

General reference

English

- *The Concise Oxford Dictionary* or *Chambers Dictionary*.

- Fowler's *Modern English Usage* – a helpful reference book for problems relating to English usage and grammar.

- Roget's *Thesaurus of English Words and Phrases* – this book lists words according to their meaning.

Information about correct forms of address will assist the secretary in ascertaining decorations, honours and qualifications, and placing them in the correct sequence. For example:

- Black's *Titles and Forms of Address*
- Debrett's *Peerage and Baronetage*
- *Who's Who*.

Travel information/guides

The secretary may find the following helpful, but up-to-date information should always be obtained from appropriate sources:

- railway and airways guides
- railway timetables
- Automobile Association (AA) and Royal Automobile Club (RAC) handbooks – these give useful information for motorists and details of hotels, etc.

Addresses and telephone numbers

Reference can be made to telephone directories and *Yellow Pages* for addresses and telephone numbers and listings of names under professions or trades.

The Post Office Directory can be used for detailed information of streets and occupiers of each house/shop, etc.

General

The following are useful:

- *Whitaker's Almanac*
- *Guide to your Local Social Services Provision*
- *Post Office Guide*
- *Voluntary Services Guide*
- *Pear's Cyclopaedia*.

Further reading

- Chambers R (2000) *Involving Patients and the Public: how to do it better*. Radcliffe Medical Press, Oxford.
- Chambers R and Boath E (2001) *Clinical Effectiveness and Clinical Governance Made Easy* (2e). Radcliffe Medical Press, Oxford.
- Debell B (1997) *Conciliation and Mediation in the NHS: a practical guide*. Radcliffe Medical Press, Oxford.
- Ellis N (ed.) (2000) *General Practitioners Handbook* (2e). Radcliffe Medical Press, Oxford.
- Ellis N and Chisholm J (1997) *Making Sense of the Red Book* (3e). Radcliffe Medical Press, Oxford.
- Haman H and Irvine S (2001) *Good People, Good Practice: a practical guide to managing personnel in the new primary care organisations*. Radcliffe Medical Press, Oxford.
- Lindsay J and Ellis N (1998) *Staff Pensions in General Practice*. Radcliffe Medical Press, Oxford.
- McGhee M (2000) *A Guide to Laboratory Investigations* (3e). Radcliffe Medical Press, Oxford.
- Robbins M and Wetherfield J (1994) *Terminology for Medical Administrators*. Radcliffe Medical Press, Oxford.

Hippocratic Oath

I swear by Apollo the physician, and Aesculapius and health and All-Heal and all the gods and goddesses, that, according to my ability and judgement, I shall keep this Oath and stipulation – to reckon him who taught me this Art equally dear to me as my parents, to share my substance with him and relieve his necessities if required, to look upon his offspring as my own brothers, and to teach them this Art, if they shall wish to learn it, without fee or stipulation, and that by precept, lecture and every other mode of instruction, I shall impart knowledge of the Art of my own sons, and those of my teachers, and to disciplines bound by stipulations and oath, according to the law of medicine but to none others. I will follow that system which, according to my judgement, I consider for the benefit of my patients and abstain from whatever is harmful for them. I shall give no deadly medicine to anyone if asked, nor suggest any such consent and in like manner I shall not advise a woman to procure abortion. With purity and holiness I shall pass my life and practise my Art. Into whatever houses I enter, I shall go into them for the benefit of the sick. Whatever I see or hear, in the life of men, which ought not to be spoken abroad, I shall not divulge, as reckoning that all such should be kept secret.

Training programmes

The following are a selection of the principal nationally validated training programmes appropriate to receptionists and secretaries working in the field of healthcare.

Radcliffe Medical Press Ltd

18 Marcham Road
Abingdon
Oxon OX14 1AA
Tel: 01235 528820

PRP *Flexible Learning for Administrative Staff in Primary Care Programmes 1, 2 and 3*
Hospital Receptionist Programmes 1 and 2
Dental Receptionist Programmes 1 and 2

These training programmes can be used to provide significant evidence and underpinning knowledge for the NVQ (Administration) Level 2. PRP and HRP certificates are awarded on satisfactory completion of courses which are also available as distance/open learning training programmes.

Healthcare Supervisory Development

A flexible learning programme designed to bridge the gap between NVQ Level 2, Administration and Level 4, Management. A National Certificate in Healthcare Supervision is awarded on satisfactory completion of the programme.

Association of Medical Secretaries, Practice Managers, Administrators and Receptionists (AMSPAR)

Tavistock House North
Tavistock Square
London WC1H 9LN
Tel: 0207 387 6005

Certificate in General Practice Reception
Advanced Certificate in General Practice Reception

Diploma in Health Service Reception (flexible methods of delivery)
Certificate in Medical Terminology
Diploma or Certificate in Medical Secretarial Studies

RSA Examinations Board

Westwood House
Westwood Way
Coventry CV4 8HS
Tel: 01203 470033

Medical Shorthand Speed Test, 80, 90, 100 wpm
Medical Audio Transcription
Medical Audio Transcription (Parts 1 and 2, Modular Award)
Medical Word Processing (Parts 1 and 2, Modular Award)

Pitman Examinations Institute

Medical Shorthand, 80, 90, 100 wpm

National Traineeship

National Traineeship is a new initiative providing an option for young people who want to continue in full-time work and train towards vocational qualifications (NVQ Level 2 – Care) in health and social care. National Traineeships provide a structured programme of work-based training and are supported by professional carers and trainers.

Medical terminology

Some components of words referring to body structures

A knowledge of these words will help you to deduce the meanings of many of the medical terms you hear and see in the course of your work.

Component of word	Pertaining to
aden	gland
angi	vessels (especially blood vessels)
arthr	joint(s)
aur	ear(s)
cardi	heart
caud	tail
cephal	head
cheil	lip(s)
chole	biliary system
cholecyst	gall-bladder
chondr	cartilage
col	colon
cyst	bladder
derm	skin
enter	intestine
fibr	fibrous tissue
gastr	stomach
gloss	tongue
haem or hem	blood
hepat	liver
hyster	uterus
labi	lips
lymph	lymphatic system
mamm, mast	breast(s)
myel	bone marrow or spinal cord
myo	muscle(s)
nephr	kidney(s)
ocul, ophthal	eye
onych	nails
orch, orchid	testes
or	mouth

os, oste	bone(s)
ot	ear(s)
pneumon	lung(s)
proct	rectum
pyel	kidney pelvis
ren	kidneys
rhin	nose
salping	uterine tubes
sial	salivary glands
spondyl	vertebra(ae)

Suffixes

Suffix	Meaning	Example	Definition
-algia	pain	arthralgia	joint pain
-ac	pertaining to	cardiac	pertaining to the heart
-al			
-ar		vascular	relating to blood vessels
-ary		coronary	pertaining to the heart
-ic	referring to	pelvic	relating to the pelvis
-ory		sensory	pertaining to feeling
-ous	denoting	cutaneous	pertaining to the skin
-aemia	blood	hyperglycaemia	high blood sugar
-cele	swelling, hernia	cystocele	hernia of the bladder
		myelocele	protrusion of spinal cord through vertebrae
-centesis	puncture	paracentesis	puncture of a cavity
		thoracocentesis	aspiration of pleural cavity
-cyte	cell	leucocyte	white blood cell
-desis	binding, fixation	arthodesis	surgical fixation of a joint
-dynia	pain	pleurodynia	pain in the intercostal muscles
-ectasis	dilation	atelectasis	abnormal dilation of bronchus or bronchi
-ectomy	removal, excision	tonsillectomy	removal of tonsils
-genic	origin	bronchogenic	originating in bronchi
-genesis	forming, producing	pathogenesis	producing disease
-gram	tracing, recording	venogram	recording (X-ray) of veins
-graphy	process of recording	arteriography	X-ray of arteries
-iasis	condition of, presence, formation of	lithiasis	formation of stones
		cholelithiasis	formation of stones in gall-bladder
-itis	inflammation	carditis	inflammation of heart

		rhinitis	inflammation of mucous membrane of nose
-logy	study of	cytology	study of cells
-malacia	softening	osteomalacia	softening of bone
-megaly	enlargement	cardiomegaly	enlargement of heart
-oid	like, resembling	osteoid	like bone
-oma	tumour	osteoma	tumour of bone
-osis	disease, abnormal condition	spondylosis	disease of spine
-pathy	disease	myelopathy	disease of spinal cord
-penia	lack of	leucopenia	deficiency of white blood cells
-phasis	ability to speak	dysphasia	difficulty in speaking
-phagia	ability to swallow	dysphagia	difficulty in swallowing
-phobia	fear of	agoraphobia	fear of open spaces
-pnoea	breath	dyspnoea	difficulty in breathing
-rrhage	a bursting out	haemorrhage	an escape of blood from the vessels
-stasis	arrest, or cessation, a halting	haemostasis	the arrest of a flow of blood
-trophy	nourishment	atrophy	to waste away
-uria	pertaining to urine	haematuria	presence of blood in urine

Prefixes

Suffix	Meaning	Example	Definition
a-	absence, lack of	amnesia	loss of memory
ab-	from, away from	abduct	move away from mid-line of body
ad-	to, towards	adduct	move towards the mid-line of body
an-	absence, lack of	anaesthesia	loss of sensation
ante-	before	antepartum	before delivery
anti-	against	antiseptic	agent used against bacteria
brady-	slow	bradycardia	slow heart beat
contra-	opposite	contralateral	opposite side
circum-	around	cirumoral	around the mouth
com-	with	compound	to mix or fuse
con-	jointed	congenital	present at birth
di-	disengage	diarthrosis	to separate from a joint
dia-	through, by means of		
ec-	out from	ectopic	not in normal place
endo	within	endometrium	lining of the uterus
exo-	outside	exogenous	produced outside

hypo-	beneath	hypotension	below normal blood pressure
infra-	under	infrapatellar	under the kneecap
inter-	between	intercostal	between the ribs
intra-	within	intracellular	within a cell
mega-	large, abnormally enlarged	megacolon	abnormally large (dilated) colon
micro-	abnormally small	microscopic	visible only with aid of microscope
onc-	pertaining to tumours	oncology	scientific study of tumours
para-	near, beside	paravertebral	beside the vertebra
peri-	around	pericardium	around the heart
pre-	forwards	prenatal	before birth
pro-	in front of	prognosis	forecast (of course of disease)
retro-	backwards	retroflexion	bending backward
sym-	beside	symphysis	growing together
syn-	along	synapse	joining of two neurones
tachy-	rapid	tachycardia	rapid heart beat
trans-	across	transurethral	through the urethra

Some of the most commonly used abbreviations

AID	artificial insemination by donor
AIDS	acquired immune deficiency syndrome
APH	antepartum haemorrhage
ASD	atrial septal defect
ASD	autistic spectrum disorders
bd	twice per day
BI	bony injury
BP	blood pressure, *British Pharmacopoeia*
CDH	congenital dislocation of the hip
CSF	cerebrospinal fluid
CNS	central nervous system
CT	computerised tomography
CAT	computerised axial tomography
CSU	catheter specimen of urine
CVP	central venous pressure
CVS	cardiovascular system
D&C	dilatation and curettage (uterine)
DLE	disseminated lupus erythematosus
DNA	did not attend (or deoxyribonucleic acid)
DS	disseminated sclerosis
DU	duodenal ulcer
D&V	diarrhoea and vomiting
DVT	deep vein thrombosis
DXRT	deep X-ray therapy
ECG	electrocardiography

EDD	expected date of delivery
ENT	ear, nose and throat
ESR	erythrocyte sedimentation rate
EUA	examination under anaesthetic
FB	foreign body
FHH	fetal heart heard
FDIU	fetal death *in utero*
GU	gastric ulcer
Hb	haemoglobin
HRT	hormone replacement therapy
IM	intramuscular
Ig	immunoglobulin
ISQ	in status quo (unchanged)
IUCD	intrauterine contraceptive device
IUD	intrauterine death or intrauterine (contraceptive) device
IV	intravenous
LB	loose body
MI	myocardial infarct
MRI	magnetic resonance imaging
MS	multiple sclerosis or mitral stenosis
MSU	midstream specimen of urine
NAD	no abnormality detected
NAI	non-accidental injury
NG	new growth
NYD	not yet diagnosed
OA	osteoarthritis
OT	occupational therapy
PET	positron emission tomography
PID	prolapsed intervertebral disc
PM	post-mortem
POP	plaster of Paris
PPH	postpartum haemorrhage
PR	per (through) the rectum
PUO	pyrexia of unknown origin
PV	per (through) the vagina
RA	rheumatoid arthritis
RBC	red blood cell
RH	rhesus factor
SMR	submucous resection of nasal septum
SOB	shortness of breath
SOL	space-occupying lesion
SOS	if necessary
SPECT	single photon emission computerised tomography
TB	tuberculosis or tubercle bacilli
tds	three times a day
THR	total hip replacement
TPR	temperature, pulse and respiration
Ts & As	tonsils and adenoids
TUR	transurethral resection (of prostate)
UTI	urinary tract infection
VD	venereal disease

VVs	varicose veins
WBC	white blood cells
WR	Wassermann reaction
XR	X-ray

Medical symbols

♀	male
♂	female
#	fracture
Δ	diagnosis
R$_x$	recipe (for prescription – 'take thou')
+ve	positive
–ve	negative
$\bar{c}$	with
$\bar{s}$	without
1/7	one day
3/7	three days
1/52	one week
1/12	one month

Abbreviations used in prescribing

Abbreviation	Latin equivalent	English meaning
aa	ana	of each the amount
ac	ante cibum	before food
bd (or bid)	bis die (bis in die)	twice daily
$\bar{c}$	cum	with
hn	hac nocte	tonight
mane	mane	in the morning
mdu	more dicta utendus	as previously directed
m et n	mane et nocte	morning and night
nocte	nocte	at night
om	omni mane	every morning
on	omni nocte	every night
pc	post cibum	after food
prn	pre re nata	whenever necessary
qds	quater die sumendum	four times a day
qid	quater in die	four times a day
sos	si opus sit	if necessary
stat	statim	immediately
td (or tid)	ter die (ter in die)	three times a day
tds	ter die sumendum	three times a day

Investigations

Digestive system

Test	Reason for test
Oral cytology	Detection of early cancer in the elderly
Oesophagoscopy (visual inspection of oesophagus)	Investigation of tumours, strictures; removal of foreign bodies
Gastroscopy (visual inspection of stomach)	Investigation of abnormalities (e.g. gastric ulcer, carcinoma)
Liver function tests (LFTs)	Liver disease; obstructive jaundice; haemolytic jaundice
Endoscopic retrograde cholangio-pancreatography (ERCP)	Detection of pancreatic cancer
Glucose tolerance tests (GTTs)	To test the patient's ability to stabilise his or her blood level
Laparoscopy (visual inspection of abdominal cavity)	Investigation of lower abdominal pain
Proctoscopy (visual inspection of anal canal and lower rectum)	Detection of haemorrhoids or growths
Colonoscopy (visual inspection of colon)	Investigation of malignant changes or for biopsy
Sigmoidoscopy (visual inspection of sigmoid colon)	Detection of growths; ulcerative colitis
Examination of faeces	Diagnosis of gastric/duodenal ulcers/carcinoma

Investigations and tests relating to haematology and blood transfusion

Test	Reason for test
Haemoglobin (Hb) estimation	Detection of abnormalities (e.g. polycythaemia, anaemia)
Red blood cell count (RBC)	
Haematocrit or packed cell volume (PCV)	Routine blood investigations for presence of abnormalities
Mean corpuscular haemoglobin (MCH)	
Mean corpuscular haemoglobin concentration (MCHC)	
Erythrocyte sedimentation rate (ESR)	A test to screen for systematic disease, or progress of disease (e.g. inflammatory and autoimmune disease, malignancy, serious infection)

White blood cell count (WBC)	Detection of disease and infection (e.g. pneumonia, leukaemia, appendicitis)
Platelet count	Detection of disease, trauma, infection, inflammation, malignancy
Clotting time	To test extrinsic clotting system in diagnosis of haemophilia, obstructive jaundice, etc.
Prothrombin ratio	Investigation of haemorrhagic disorders, liver disease
Paul Bunnell	To diagnose infective mononucleosis (glandular fever)
Monospot	To diagnose infective mononucleosis (glandular fever)
Rose–Waaler (RA)	To diagnose rheumatoid arthritis
Latex fixation test	To diagnose rheumatoid arthritis
Antinuclear factor/antibody (ANF/ANA)	To diagnose systemic lupus erythematosus

Bacterial tests on blood

Widal reaction (WR)	Diagnosis of typhoid/paratyphoid and brucellosis
VDRL	Diagnosis of venereal disease
TPHA	Diagnosis of venereal disease
WR	Diagnosis of venereal disease
GCFT	Diagnosis of venereal disease
Guthrie's test	Estimation of blood level of phenylketonuria (PKU) in babies

Musculoskeletal system

Disorders of bones and joints give rise to pain, deformity, swelling of bone and tissues, limitation of movement and secondary muscle wasting.

X-ray investigation is of value in diagnosis and assessment of the response to treatment. Bone scanning is increasingly being used for detection of malignant conditions in bone.

Test	Reason for test
Arthroscopy (visual inspection of knee joint)	Diagnosis of disease/injury to interior of joint
Electromyography	Detection of muscular disorders (e.g. muscular dystrophy, myasthenia gravis and myotonia)
Myelography	Detection of spinal lesions (e.g. tumours and prolapsed intervertebral disc)
Radiculography	Similar procedure to myelography, used to investigate the lumbosacral nerve roots

(see also Miscellaneous investigations)

Cardiovascular system

Test	Reason for test
Blood pressure (BP)	To detect disease Hypertension – abnormally high blood pressure Hypotension – abnormally low blood pressure
Angio-cardiography (injection of dye through catheter enabling X-ray of heart structure)	Detection of abnormalities of the heart and blood vessels
Electrocardiography (ECG) (recording of electrical activity of the heart)	To investigate heart disorders (e.g. coronary thrombosis, heart block)
Echocardiography	Diagnosis of valvular disease and pericardial effusion

Respiratory system

Test	Reason for test
Rhinoscopy (examination of interior of nose)	Removal of tissue for histology, or swab taken for bacteriology
Laryngoscopy	Examination of vocal cords, larynx and epiglottis, for growths and infections
Bronchoscopy (visual inspection of bronchi)	Diagnosis of growths; tissue removal for biopsy
Sputum examination	Examination of sputum for blood, parasites, etc.
Pleural fluid	Detection of malignancy, chest injury, emphysema, heart failure

Lung function tests

Vital capacity of lungs (maximum amount of air which can be expired)	Measurement of amount of air expired by a patient – diminished in lung disease
Wright's peak-flow meter	Detection of lung disease

Nervous system

Test	Reason for test
Lumbar puncture	Examination of cerebrospinal fluid (CSF) and diagnosis of certain diseases of nervous system

Romberg's sign	Test for co-ordination, used in diagnosis of multiple sclerosis, cerebral tumour, etc.
Kernig's sign	Diagnosis of meningitis, cerebral haemorrhage or meningism
Electroencephalogram (EEG)	Investigation of epileptic conditions and location of cerebral lesions
Electromyogram (EMG) (recording of electrical activity in a muscle)	Investigation of disease
Knee jerk	Detection of disease of nervous system

Pupil reflexes

Reaction to light	Detection of diseases of central nervous system

Eye tests

Optic discs	Detection of disease of central nervous system
Snellen's test	Measurement of extent of field of vision
Refraction tests	To correct defective vision by prescription of correct lens

Hearing tests

Audiometric tests	Determination of degree and type of hearing
Weber's test (tuning fork)	To distinguish between middle-ear and nerve deafness
Rinne's test	Detection of middle-ear deafness
Auriscopy (visual examination of middle ear)	Detection of infection and disease

Urinary system

Test	Reason for test
Routine laboratory examination	Detection of urinary infections, pyelonephritis, haematuria (blood in urine)
Mid-stream urine specimen (MSU)	Nephritis, presence of parasites – tropical disease

Test for protein	Presence of protein in urine (albuminuria)
Test for sugar	Presence of sugar in urine (glycosuria)
Test for ketones	Presence of ketones in urine (ketonuria)
Test for blood	Presence of blood in urine (haematuria)

Renal efficiency tests

Blood urea	Impairment of renal function
Urea clearance test	To indicate extent of kidney damage
Cystoscopy (visual inspection of bladder)	Detection of disease of bladder; for biopsy of tissue/tumour
Intravenous pyelogram (IVP)	To test renal function; to demonstrate hydronephrosis, renal calculi, hydronephroma, etc.
Renal biopsy	Specimen sent for histology

Pregnancy tests

Oestriol examination	Assessment of both placental and fetal function
Toxaemia of pregnancy	Urine tested for protein – to confirm condition
Amniocentesis	Estimation of fetal maturity; detection of fetal defects, etc.
Cervical smear	Early diagnosis of cancer; detection of infection and other conditions
Vaginal swab	To detect cause of vaginal discharge

Endocrine glands

Test	Reason for test
Thyroid function tests (TFTs)	Assessment of functioning of thyroid glands
Protein-bound iodine (PBI)	Measurement of thyroid function

X-ray investigations

Test	Reason for test
Barium swallow	Detection of lesions of oesophagus; demonstration of hiatus hernia
Barium meal	Detection of lesions of stomach and duodenum
Barium meal with follow-through	Detection of lesions of small and large intestines
Barium enema	Detection of disease and obstruction of the bowel
Double-contrast radiography	Detection of small changes in gastric mucosa (e.g. early carcinoma)
Cholecystography	To demonstrate presence of gallstones
Intravenous cholangiogram	To demonstrate bile duct obstruction due to growth or stones
Arthrogram	To outline joint cavity
Bone scan	Detection of secondary tumours
Angiography	Demonstration of obstruction, aneurysm or abnormal course (of blood vessel)
Aortogram	Angiogram of aorta
Arteriogram	Angiogram of arteries
Venogram	Angiogram of veins
Bronchography	Diagnosis of bronchiectasis and other bronchial abnormalities
Lung scan	Demonstration of tumours
Mammography	Detection of early malignancy of breast
Myelogram	Examination of spinal cord for obstruction and other defects
Encephalogram	Detection of cerebral tumours
Ventriculogram	To confirm cerebral tumour

Skin tests

Mantoux test	Skin test for sensitivity to TB by dilute intradermal injection of tuberculin
Heaf test	Similar to Mantoux, but using multiple-puncture technique
Kveim test	Intradermal injection to diagnose sarcoidosis

Miscellaneous investigations

Radiography

X-rays are one of the most frequently requested investigations used by physicians. They are painless unless used in conjunction with a contrast medium, which may cause discomfort. They are also quick and easy to perform, but may be frightening for the patient.

X-rays are a form of electromagnetic energy of a short wavelength which have the ability to penetrate tissues.

Plain X-rays are commonly performed on the chest, the abdomen, the skull and limbs in order to study bones for bone disease, fractures, etc. Contrast media may be used to visualise soft tissues and organs.

Ultrasonography (ultrasound)

Ultrasound is a non-invasive diagnostic procedure used to view body structures. It is convenient, safe and a comparatively inexpensive investigation. It does not use ionising radiation and is therefore safer than radiography. Ultrasound examinations are performed on the following structures:

* the brain – electroencephalography

* the arteries and veins

* the heart – echocardiography

* the kidney, liver and pelvis.

In obstetrics, the main use of ultrasonography is to demonstrate fetal size and growth, and the position of the placenta.

Computed tomography

Computed tomography (CT) scanning is an X-ray technique which uses a computer to reconstruct an image of a layer of tissue in the body. The CT scanner can image the three main cavities of the body (head, thorax and abdomen). It is mainly used for detecting lesions such as tumours and cysts in the body.

A second-generation CT system has evolved which produces three-dimensional images of the body. These latest three-dimensional images allow doctors to examine, for example, a person's brain as if it were being held in their hands.

Nuclear magnetic resonance imaging (NMRI)

This form of investigation is now widely used in medicine, and is often referred to as MRI. It uses radio-frequency radiation in the presence of a magnetic field to produce anatomical sections of the human body.

It is a non-invasive technique, it does not use ionising radiation, and it penetrates the structures of the body. In contrast with CT scanning, MRI can provide images in any anatomical plane.

Radioisotope scanning

A radioactive isotope is an unstable isotope which decays or disintegrates, emitting radiation or energy as it does so. The energy source is inside the patient and is given either orally or intravenously.

Radioisotopic scans are performed in order to detect malfunction or abnormalities of bones, lungs, brain, heart, kidneys, gall-bladder, spleen and endocrine glands.

Thermography

This is a technique which measures and records heat energy from the skin surface. It is non-invasive and causes no discomfort. Films are taken in much the same way as a photograph. Plates with these films are placed on the skin and changes of skin temperature are reflected on a colour map.

Thermography is mainly used to detect lesions of the breast, to evaluate drug therapy, and to diagnose spinal root compression, and it may be used to assess the progress of wound healing.

Tomography

This is a technique in which a single layer of tissue is examined. This is achieved by blurring the image of the tissues above and below the layer of tissue to be studied when the X-ray is taken.

Fluoroscopy

Fluoroscopy enables the function of organs to be directly visualised in motion on a fluorescent screen (e.g. the heart beat, movement of the diaphragm and motility of the gastrointestinal tract can be observed and recorded).

Immunisation schedules

Recommended immunisations for children

The schedule below is currently recommended by the Department of Health.

When is the immunisation due?	Which immunisation?	Type
At two months	• Polio	By mouth
	• Hib • Diphtheria • Tetanus • Whooping cough (pertussis)	One injection
	• Meningitis C	One injection
At three months	• Polio	By mouth
	• Hib • Diphtheria • Tetanus • Whooping cough	One injection
	• Meningitis C	One injection
At four months	• Polio	By mouth
	• Hib • Diphtheria • Tetanus • Whooping cough	One injection
	Meningitis C	One injection
At 12 to 15 months	• Measles • Mumps • Rubella	One injection

The Department of Health advises that children should not be given separate measles, mumps and rubella vaccines in place of MMR, since there is no evidence of benefit and a clear risk of harm from following such a practice.

Cont

3 to 5 years (usually before the child starts school)	• Measles • Mumps • Rubella	One injection
	• Diphtheria • Tetanus	One injection
	• Polio	By mouth
10 to 14 years (sometimes shortly after birth)	• BCG (tuberculosis)	Skin test followed by one injection
School leavers **13 to 18 years**	• Diphtheria • Tetanus	One injection
	• Polio	By mouth

© 2001 Crown Copyright

Recommended immunisations for adults

Disease	Frequency	Method
Tetanus toxoid	Booster every 10 years	One injection, or three at monthly intervals for those previously unvaccinated
Polio	Booster every 10 years until age 40 years	By mouth (OPV)
For at-risk groups		
Influenza	Annually (especially for the elderly)	Injection
Hepatitis B	Booster every 3–5 years	Injections (in first instance, three over 6 months, followed by blood test)

Vaccinations for foreign travel

Travellers to hot climates and developing countries should be given immunisations and anti-malarial advice according to up-to-date recommendations which can be found in the *Pulse* and *MIMS* charts which are published monthly, and the patient's previous immunisation status.

Incubation periods of some infectious diseases

The incubation period is the interval between the time of primary infection or contact with an infected person and the appearance of the disease. The following information is only a guide, as in some instances some of the diseases have been found to have an incubation period outside the stated range.

Disease or causative organism	Incubation period
Amoebic dysentery	1–4 weeks
Bacillus cereus enteritis	1–5 hours
Botulism	2 hours – 8 days (usually 12–36 hours)
Brucellosis	1–8 weeks (usually 2–3 weeks)
Campylobacter enteritis	1–11 days (usually 2–5 days)
Chicken-pox	10–21 days (usually 14–15 days)
Cholera	2–48 hours
Dysentery	1–7 days (usually 1–3 days)
German measles (rubella)	14–21 days
Infective jaundice (hepatitis A)	14–42 days
Hepatitis B	42 days – 6 months
Lassa fever	3–17 days
Legionnaire's disease	2–10 days
Leptospirosis	4–19 days (usually 7–12 days)
Malaria	8–25 days
Measles	7–21 days (usually 10–14 days)
Mumps	12–28 days (usually 16–18 days)
Polio	10–15 days
Rabies	2 weeks–5 years (usually 20–90 days)
Salmonella enteritis	6–72 hours
Scarlet fever	2–5 days
Typhoid fever	7–21 days
Whooping cough	5–21 days
Yellow fever	3–6 days

Abbreviations of qualifying degrees and further qualifications

ABPN	Association of British Psychiatric Nurses
AIHA	Association of the Institute of Hospital Administration
AIMLS	Association of the Institute of Medical Laboratory Sciences
BAc	Bachelor of Acupuncture
BAO	Bachelor of the Art of Obstetrics
BC, BCh, BChir	Bachelor of Surgery
BM	Bachelor of Medicine
BS, ChB, CChir	Bachelor of Surgery
BSc	Bachelor of Science
BSc (Soc Sci Nurs)	Bachelor of Nursing
CCFP	Certificate of the College of Family Practitioners
ChD	Doctor of Surgery
CM, ChM	Master of Surgery
CPH	Certificate in Public Health
CTCM&H	Certificate in Tropical Community Medicine and Hygiene
DA	Diploma in Anaesthetics
DavMed	Diploma in Aviation Medicine
DCCH	Diploma in Child and Community Health
DCH	Diploma in Child Health
DCh	Doctor of Surgery
DCP	Diploma in Clinical Pathology
DCPath	Diploma of the College of Pathologists
DCR	Diploma of the College of Radiologists
DDR	Diploma in Diagnostic Radiology
DDS	Doctor of Dental Surgery
DFM	Diploma in Forensic Medicine
DGM	Diploma in Geriatric Medicine
DHyg	Doctor of Hygiene
DIH	Diploma in Industrial Health
Dip GU Med	Diploma in Genitourinary Medicine
DLO	Diploma in Laryngology and Otology
Dip Med Rehab	Diploma in Medical Rehabilitation
DM	Doctor of Medicine

DMR	Diploma in Medical Radiology
DMRT	Diploma in Medical Radiotherapy
DN	Diploma in Nursing, District Nurse
DO	Diploma in Ophthalmology
DObstRCOG	Diploma in Obsterics of the Royal College of Obstetricians and Gynaecologists
DOMS	Diploma in Ophthalmological Medicine and Surgery
DPH	Diploma in Public Health
DPM	Diploma in Psychological Medicine
DR	Diploma in Radiology
DrAc	Doctor of Acupuncture
DSc	Doctor of Science
DTM&H	Diploma in Tropical Medicine and Hygiene
En(G)	Enrolled Nurse (General)
En(M)	Enrolled Nurse (Mental)
FCGP	Fellow of the College of General Practitioners
FCOphth	Fellow of the College of Ophthalmology
FCPath	Fellow of the College of Pathologists
FDS	Fellow of Dental Surgery
FFARCS	Fellow of the Faculty of Anaesthetists of the Royal College of Surgeons
FFHom	Fellow of the Faculty of Homeopathy
FFR	Fellow of the Faculty of Radiologists
FIBiol	Fellow of the Institute of Biology
FICS	Fellow of the International College of Surgeons
FLCO	Fellow of the London College of Osteopathy
FPS	Fellow of the Pharmaceutical Society
FRC Anaesth	Fellow of the Royal College of Anaesthetists
FRCGP	Fellow of the Royal College of General Practitioners
FRCN	Fellow of the Royal College of Nursing
FRCOG	Fellow of the Royal College of Obstetricians and Gynaecologists
FRCP	Fellow of the Royal College of Physicians of London
FRCPE	Fellow of the Royal College of Physicians of Edinburgh (may also be written as FRCPEd, FRCPEdin)
FRCPS	Fellow of the Royal College of Physicians and Surgeons
FRCPath	Fellow of the Royal College of Pathologists
FRCPsych	Fellow of the Royal College of Psychiatrists
FRCR	Fellow of the Royal College of Radiologists
FRCS	Fellow of the Royal College of Surgeons of England
FRCSE	Fellow of the Royal College of Surgeons of Edinburgh
FRIPHH	Fellow of the Royal Institute of Public Health and Hygiene
FRS	Fellow of the Royal Society
FRSH	Fellow of the Royal Society of Health
HVCert	Health Visitors Certificate
LAH	Licentiate of Apothecaries Hall, Dublin
LDS	Licentiate in Dental Surgery
LM	Licentiate in Midwifery
LRCP	Licentiate of the Royal College of Physicians
LSA	Licentiate of the Society of Apothecaries
MAO	Master of the Art of Obstetrics

MB	Bachelor of Medicine
MB ChB	Bachelor of Medicine Bachelor of Surgery
MC, MCh, MChir	Master of Surgery
MChD	Master of Dental Surgery
MChOrth	Master of Orthopaedic Surgery
MClinPsychol	Master of Clinical Psychology
McommH	Master of Community Health
MCPath	Member of College of Pathology
MCPS	Member of College of Physicians and Surgeons
MD	Doctor of Medicine
MDS	Master of Dental Surgery
MFCP	Member of the Faculty of Community Physicians
MFHom	Member of the Faculty of Homeopathy
MHyg	Master of Hygiene
MIH	Master of Industrial Health
MLCOM	Member of the London College of Osteopathic Medicine
MMed	Master of Medicine
MMSA	Master of Midwifery of Society of Apothecaries
MO&G	Master of Obstetrics and Gynaecology
MOH	Medical Officer of Health
MPH	Master of Public Health
MPS	Member of the Pharmaceutical Society
MPsy	Master of Psychiatry
MPsychMed	Master of Psychological Medicine
MRad(D)	Master of Radiodiagnosis
MRad(T)	Master of Radiotherapy
MRCGP	Member of the Royal College of General Practitioners
MRCOG	Member of the Royal College of Obstetricians and Gynaecologists
MRCP	Member of the Royal College of Physicians
MRCPath	Member of the Royal College of Pathologists
MRCPsych	Member of the Royal College of Psychiatrists
MRCS	Member of the Royal College of Surgeons of England
MS	Master of Surgery
MSR(R)	Member of the Society of Radiography (Radiography)
MSR(T)	Member of the Society of Radiography (Radiotherapy)
RCM	Royal College of Midwives
RCN	Royal College of Nursing
RGN	Registered General Nurse
SEN	State Enrolled Nurse
SRN	State Registered Nurse
SRP	State Registered Physiotherapist

Other medical abbreviations (including job titles, organisations and non-clinical terms)

AHCPA	Association of Health Centres and Practice Administrators
AMSPAR	Association of Medical Secretaries, Practice Managers, Administrators and Receptionists
BACUP	British Association of Cancer-United Families and their families and friends
BMA	British Medical Association
BMJ	*British Medical Journal*
BNF	*British National Formulary*
BP	*British Pharmacopoeia*
BPC	British Pharmaceutical Codex
BRCS	British Red Cross Society
CDSR	Cochrane Database of Systematic Reviews
CEM	cost-effectiveness-based medical decision making
CHC	Community Health Council
CMB	Central Midwives Board
CME	continuing medical education
CNO	Chief Nursing Officer
CPA	Care Programme Approach
CRDC	Central R & D Committee
CRES	cash-releasing efficiency savings
DDA	Dangerous Drugs Act
DN	District Nurse
DoH	Department of Health
DSS	Department of Social Security
EBM	evidence-based medicine
ECHR	European Convention on Human Rights
ECR	extra-contractual referral
EDI	electronic data interchange
EPR	electronic paper record
FPA	Family Planning Association
GDP	General Dental Practitioner
GMC	General Medical Council
GMSC	General Medical Services Committee
GMP	General Medical Practitioner
HAZ	Health Action Zone
HCHS	hospital and community health services
HIMP	Health Improvement Programme
HTA	Health Technology Assessment
HV	Health Visitor
IHSM	Institute of Health Services Management
ILA	Independent Learning Account
IMA	Independent Medical Adviser
LMG	Local Medical Committee
MAAG	Medical Audit Advisory Group
MDU	Medical Defence Union

MIMS	*Monthly Index of Medical Specialities*
MPS	Medical Protection Society
MRC	Medical Research Council
MSW	Medical Social Worker
NAHAT	National Association of Health Authorities and Trusts
NBTS	National Blood Transfusion Service
NCCHTA	National Co-ordinating Centre for Health Technology Assessment
NHS	National Health Service
NICE	National Institute for Clinical Excellence
OCDMA	Oncology Data Managers Association
OT	Occupational Therapist
PACT	Prescribing Analyses and Costs
PALS	Patient Advocacy and Liaison Service
PAM	professions allied to medicine
PCG	Primary Care Group
PCLM	Primary Care Liaison Manager
PCT	Primary Care Trust
PGEA	Postgraduate Educational Allowance
PRINCE	PRojects IN Controlled Environment
QALY	Quality-Adjusted Life Year
QCA	Qualifications Curriculum Authority
RCGP	Royal College of General Practitioners
RHA	Regional Health Authority
SHO	Senior House Officer
SI	Systeme International (units)
ST	Speech Therapist
TQM	Total Quality Management
UKCC	United Kingdom Council for Nursing Midwifery and Health Visiting
WHO	World Health Organisation

Useful addresses

Association of Community Health Councils
362 Euston Road
London NW1
Tel: 0207 388 4874

Association of Health Centre and Practice Administrators (AHCPA)
c/o Royal College of General Practitioners
14 Princes Gate
London SW7 1PU
Tel: 0207 581 3232

Association of Medical Secretaries, Practice Administrators and Receptionists (AMSPAR)
Tavistock House North
Tavistock Square
London WC1H 9LN
Tel: 0207 387 6005

British Medical Association (BMA)
BMA House
Tavistock Square
London WC1H 9JP
Tel: 0207 387 4499

Department of Social Security (DSS)
Eileen House
Elephant and Castle
London SE1 6BY
Tel: 0207 703 6380

General Medical Council (GMC)
178 Great Portland Street
London W1N 6JE
Tel: 0207 580 7642

GP Computer Centre
75 York Road
London SE1 7NT
Tel: 0207 620 0901

Health and Safety Executive
Broad Lane
Sheffield SE3 7HQ
Tel: 0114 289 2000

Health Service Commissioner (Ombudsman) for England
Church House
Great Smith Street
London SW1P 3BW
Tel: 0207 276 2035 or 3000
(investigates complaints about health authorities in England)

Health Services Commissioner for Scotland
2nd Floor
11 Melville Crescent
Edinburgh EH3 7LU
Tel: 0131 225 7465

Health Services Commissioner for Wales
4th Floor
Pearl Assurance House
Greyfriars Road
Cardiff CF1 3AG
Tel: 01222 394621

Hospital Consultants and Specialists Association
The Old Court House
London Road
Ascot
Berks SL5 7EN
Tel: 01344 25052

Institute of Health and Care Development
St Bartholomew's Court
18 Christmas Street
Bristol BS1 5BT
Tel: 0207 929 1029

Institute of Health Services Management (IHSM)
7–10 Chandos Street
London W1M 9DE
Tel: 0207 460 7654

King's Fund
11–13 Cavendish Square
London W1M 0AN
Tel: 0207 307 2400

Medical Defence Union
3 Devonshire Place
London W1N 2EA
Tel: 0207 202 1500

Medical Protection Society
50 Hallam Street
London W1N 6DE
Tel: 0207 637 0541

National Association of Health Authorities and Trusts (NAHAT)
26 Chapter Street
London SW1P 4ND
Tel: 0207 233 7388

National Council for Vocational Qualifications
222 Euston Road
London NW1 2BZ
Tel: 0207 387 3611

Royal College of General Practitioners
14 Princes Gate
Hyde Park
London SW7 1PU
Tel: 0207 581 3232

Royal College of Obstetricians and Gynaecologists
27 Sussex Place
Regents Park
London NW1 4RG
Tel: 0207 262 5425

Royal College of Nursing (UK)
Henrietta Place
London W1M 0AB
Tel: 0207 580 2646

Royal College of Pathologists
2 Carlton House Terrace
London SW1Y 5AF
Tel: 0207 930 5861

Royal College of Physicians
11 St Andrew's Place
London NW1 4LE
Tel: 0207 935 1174

Royal College of Physicians of Edinburgh
9 Queen Street
Edinburgh EH2 1JQ
Tel: 0131 225 7324

Royal College of Physicians and Surgeons of Glasgow
232–242 St Vincent Street
Glasgow G2 5RJ
Tel: 0141 221 6072

Royal College of Psychiatrists
17 Belgrave Square
London SW1X 8PG
Tel: 0207 235 2351

Royal College of Surgeons of Edinburgh
Nicolson Street
Edinburgh EH8 9DW
Tel: 0131 556 6206

Royal College of Surgeons of England
35–43 Lincoln's Inn Fields
London WC2A 3PN
Tel: 0207 405 3474

Royal Society of Medicine
1 Wimpole Street
London W1M 8AE
Tel: 0207 408 2119

RSA Examinations Board
Westwood Way
Coventry CV4 8HS
Tel: 01203 470033

Statutory organisations

(including addresses and main functions)

This includes a selection of statutory bodies (government funded) which will be of interest and use to receptionists and secretaries working in healthcare, as their activities are related to health matters in the UK.

Audit Commission
1 Vincent Square, London SW1P 2PN. Tel: 0207 828 1212.
The Audit Commission promotes studies to ascertain efficiency, effectiveness and economy in local government and the NHS, and appoints auditors to the latter.

Clinical Standards Advisory Group
Room 19, Wellington House, 133–155 Waterloo Road, London SE1 8UG.
Tel: 0207 972 4918.
The Clinical Standards Advisory Group advises the NHS and its ministers on standards of clinical care of patients, and access to and availability of services.

Common Services Agency for the Scottish Health Service
Trinity Park House, South Trinity Road, Edinburgh EH5 3SE. Tel: 0131 552 6255.
This organisation provides the NHS in Scotland with a range of services.

General Medical Council (GMC)
178 Great Portland Street, London WIN 6JE. Tel: 0207 580 7642.
The GMC is the regulatory body for the medical profession. It also sets educational and ethical standards, and has the power to discipline doctors if necessary.

Health and Safety Commission and Health and Safety Executive
2 Southwark Bridge Road, London SE1 9HS. Tel: 0207 717 6000.

The above organisations are both responsible for securing the health, safety and welfare of people and protecting the public against risks to health or safety from work activities.

Health Education Authority
88 Trevelyan House, 30 Great Peter Street, London SWIP 2HW.
Tel: 0207 222 5300.
The Health Education Authority advises health departments on health education issues. The Health Education Board for Scotland (Woodburn House, Canaan Lane, Edinburgh EH10 4SG. Tel: 0131 447 8044) and the Health Promotion Authority for Wales (Ffynnon-las Ty Glas Avenue, Llanishen, Cardiff CF4 5DZ. Tel: 01222 752222) have a similar function.

Health Service Commissioner (Ombudsman)
11th Floor, Millbank Tower, Millbank, London SE1P 4QP. Tel: 0207 276 2035.
The Ombudsman investigates complaints about services provided by the NHS, and regularly reports to Parliament.

Medical Research Council (MRC)
20 Park Crescent, London W1N 4AL. Tel: 0207 636 5542.
The MRC promotes medical and related biological research to objectively improve healthcare. It also provides grants to individual scientists.

Medicines Control Agency (MCA)
Market Towcesters, Nine Elms Lane, London SE8 5NQ. Tel: 0207 273 0393.
The MCA is an executive agency of the Department of Health and ensures that branded and non-branded medicines in the UK meet the required quality and safety standards, thus safeguarding public health. It also applies the standards set out in the Medicines Act and the legislative criteria of the European Community.

Mental Health Act Commission
Maid Marian House, Houndsgate, Nottingham NG1 6BG. Tel: 0115 943 7000.
The Mental Health Commission is responsible for protecting the interests of patients who are detained under the Mental Health Act in England and Wales. Scotland and Ireland have their own separate regulations.

Mental Welfare Commission for Scotland
Argyle House, 3 Lady Lawson Street, Edinburgh EH3 9SH. Tel: 0131 222 6111.
The Commission has the same responsibilities for Scotland as the Mental Health Act Commission does for England and Wales.

National Audit Office (NAO)
157–197 Buckingham Palace Road, Victoria, London SW1W 9SP.
Tel: 0207 798 7000.
The NAO is accountable to Parliament. It audits all public expenditure (NHS and government expediture), and reports that money has been spent for the purpose intended and is accounted for.

National Blood Authority (NBA)
Oak House, Reeds Crescent, Watford WD1 1QH. Tel: 01923 486800.
The NBA was created in 1993 to manage all NHS blood services. It manages all regional transfusion services, ensures that blood and blood product supplies meet defined criteria, and that a high-quality, cost-effective supply of both blood and blood products is available to meet national requirements (this requires approximately two million donors).

NHS Health Advisory Service (HAS)
Sutherland House, 29–37 Brighton Road, Sutton SM2 5AN. Tel: 0208 642 6421.
The HAS is an independent advisory organisation which reports to Parliament. It is responsible for improving the management of the delivery of patient care services, with special emphasis on services to the elderly, the mentally ill and those who misuse drug substances.

Northern Ireland Central Services Agency for Health and Social Services
25–27 Adelaide Street, Belfast BT2 8FH. Tel: 01232 334431.
This agency provides a range of services to the Health and Social Services Boards and to family doctors.

Prescription Pricing Authority
Bridge House, 152 Pilgrim Street, Newcastle upon Tyne NE1 2SN.
Tel: 0191 232 5371.
The Prescription Pricing Authority calculates and makes payments to dispensing doctors and pharmacists in England for NHS prescriptions dispensed. They also provide information on dispensing and prescribing to health service authorities.

Public Health Laboratory Services (PHLS)
61 Colindale Avenue, London NW9 5DF. Tel: 0208 200 1295. (Headquarters Office).
The PHLS provides facilities for the prevention and diagnosis of communicable and infectious diseases. The headquarters in Colindale provide the site of the Laboratory and Communicable Diseases Surveillance Centre and the Central Public Health Laboratory. There are approximately 50 laboratories in England and Wales, which are led by the Colindale-based laboratory.

Standing Medical Advisory Committee and Standing Nursing and Midwifery Advisory Committee
Department of Health, Room 919, Wellington House, 135–155 Waterloo Road, London SE1 8UG. Tel: 0207 972 4919.

Standing Pharmaceutical Advisory Committee
Department of Health, Room 301, Richmond House, 79 Whitehall,
London SW1A 2NS. Tel: 0207 210 6117.
These three committees advise health ministers in England and Wales on matters relating to the medical, nursing, midwifery and pharmaceutical services.

Standing Committee on Postgraduate Medical and Dental Education (SCOPME)
1 Park Square, West London NW1 41J. Tel: 0207 935 3916.
SCOPME gives advice to the Secretary of State on continuing and postgraduate medical and dental education. There are separate councils for Scotland, Northern Ireland and Wales.

United Kingdom Central Council for Nursing, Midwifery and Health Visiting (UKCC)
23 Portland Place, London W1B 4JT. Tel: 0207 637 7181.
The UKCC is a regulatory body which maintains the professional registers of nurses, midwives and health visitors, and sets standards of conduct and education for the nursing profession.

United Kingdom Transplant Support Service Authority
Fox Den Road, Stoke Gifford, Bristol BS12 6RR. Tel: 0117 975 7575.
This special health authority provides support services for the matching, allocation and distribution of donor organs for transplant.

Information and support groups

Addresses for other information and support groups can be found in the *Voluntary Agencies Directory* published by NCVO Publications, National Council for Voluntary Organisations, Regent's Wharf, 8 All Saints Street, London N1 9RL. Tel: 0207 713 6161. Telephone helpline numbers can be found in the *Telephone Helpline Directory* published by the Telephone Helplines Association, 4 Dean's Court, St Paul's Churchyard, London EC4V 5AA. Tel: 0207 248 3388.

Accident prevention in the home

Child Helpline Trust, Clarkes Court, 18–20 Farringdon Lane, London EC1R 3HA. Tel: 0207 608 3828.

Royal Society for the Prevention of Accidents, Edgbaston Park, 353 Bristol Road, Birmingham B5 7ST. Tel: 0121 248 2000.

Ageing

Age Concern England, Astral House, 268 London Road, Norbury, London SW16 4ER. Tel: 0208 765 7200.

AIDS

National Aids Helpline. Tel: 0800 555777.
Information Leaflets. Tel: 0800 567123.

London Lighthouse, 111–117 Lancaster Road, London W11 1QT. Tel: 0207 792 1200.

Communicable Diseases Surveillance Centre (PHLS), 61 Colindale Avenue, London NW9 5BQ. Tel: 0208 200 6868.

Alcohol-related problems

Alcoholics Anonymous, PO Box 1, Stonebow House, Stonebow, York YO1 2NJ. Tel: 01904 644026.

Alcohol Concern, Waterbridge House, 32–36 Loman Street, London SE1 OEE. Tel: 0207 928 7377.

Scottish Council on Alcohol, 166 Buchanan Street, Glasgow G1 2NH. Tel: 0141 333 9677.

Alzheimer's disease

Alzheimer's Disease Society, Second Floor, Gordon House, 10 Greencoat Place, London SW1P 1PH. Tel: 0207 308 0808.

Ankylosing spondylitis

National Association for Ankylosing Spondylitis, PO Box 179, Mayfield, East Sussex TN20 6ZL. Tel: 01435 873527.

Arthritis

Arthritis Care, 18 Stephenson Way, London NW1 2HD. Tel: 0207 916 1500. Helpline: 0800 289170.

ASH (Action on Smoking and Health)

ASH, 109 Gloucester Place, London W1H 4EJ. Tel: 0207 035 3519.

Asthma

National Asthma Campaign, Providence House, Providence Place, London N1 ONT. Tel: 0207 226 2260.

Autism

National Autistic Society, 276 Willesden Lane, London NW2 5RB. Tel: 0208 451 1114.

Backache

National Back Pain Association, 16 Elmtree Road, Teddington TW11 8TD. Tel: 0208 977 5474.

Blindness

Royal National Institute for the Blind, 234 Great Portland Street, London W1N 6AA. Tel: 0207 388 1255.

Blood transfusion

National Blood Authority, Oak House, Reeds Crescent, Watford WD1 1QH. Tel: 01923 486800.

Brain injuries

Headway, National Head Injuries Association, 4 King Edward Street, Nottingham NG1 1EW. Tel: 0115 924 0800.

Breast cancer care

Breast Cancer Care, Kiln House, 210 New King's Road, London SW6 4NZ. Tel: 0500 245345.

Brittle bone disease

Brittle Bone Society, 30 Guthrie Street, Dundee DD1 5BS. Tel: 01382 204446.

Cancer

Marie Curie Cancer Care, 28 Belgrave Square, London SW1X 8OG. Tel: 0207 235 3325.

Macmillan Cancer Relief, Anchor House, 15–19 Britten Street, London SW3 3TZ. Tel: 0207 351 7511.

BACUP, 3 Bath Place, Rivington Street, London EC2A 3JR. Tel: 0207 696 9003.

Carers

Carers National Association, 25 Glasshouse Yard, London EC1A 4JS. Tel: 0207 490 8818.

Women's Royal Voluntary Service, 234–244 Stockwell Road, London SW9 9SP. Tel: 0207 416 0146.

Care services

Counsel and Care, Twyman House, 16 Bonny Street, London NW1 9PG. Tel: 0207 267 6877.

Cerebral palsy

SCOPE, 6 Market Road, London N7 9PW. Tel: 0207 636 9876.

Capability Scotland, 2 Corstorphine Road, Edinburgh EH12 6HP. Tel: 0131 337 9876.

Child adoption

British Agencies for Adoption and Fostering (BAAF), Skyline House, 200 Union Street, London SE1. Tel: 0207 593 2000.

Parent-to-Parent Information on Adoptive Services (PPIAS),
Lower Boddington, Daventry, Northants NN11 6YB.

Childbirth

National Childbirth Trust, Alexandra House, Oldham Terrace, Acton,
London W3 6NH. Tel: 0208 992 6637.

Children

**Action for Sick Children (National Association for the Welfare of Children in
Hospital),** Argyle House, 29–31 Euston Road, London NW1 2SD.
Tel: 0207 833 2041.

National Society for the Prevention of Cruelty to Children (NSPCC), NSPCC
National Centre, 42 Curtain Road, London EC2A 3NH. Tel: 0207 825 2500.

Coeliac disease

Coeliac Society of the United Kingdom, PO Box 220, High Wycombe,
Bucks HP11 2HY. Tel: 01494 437278.

Colitis and Crohn's disease

National Association for Colitis and Crohn's Disease, PO Box 205, St Albans,
Herts. Tel: 01727 844296.

Colostomy

British Colostomy Association, 15 Station Road, Reading, Berks RG1 1LG.
Tel: 0118 939 1537.

Coronary heart disease

Coronary Prevention Group, Plantation House, Suite 514 D & M,
31–35 Fenchurch Street, London EC3M 3NN. Tel: 0207 626 4844.

Cystic fibrosis

Cystic Fibrosis Trust, 11 London Road, Bromley, Kent BR1 1BY.
Tel: 0208 464 7211.

Deafness

Royal National Institute for Deaf People, 19–23 Featherstone Street,
London EC1Y 8SL. Tel: 0207 296 8000.

Sense (National Deaf, Blind and Rubella Association), 11–13 Clifton Terrace,
Finsbury Park, London N4 3RS. Tel: 0207 272 7774.

Sense in Scotland, Fifth Floor, 45 Pinnieston Street, Clydeway Centre, Glasgow
G3 8JU. Tel: 0141 564 2444.

National Deaf Children's Society, 15 Dufferin Street, London EC1Y 8UR.
Tel: 0207 250 0123.

Dermatitis

National Eczema Society, 163 Eversholt Street, London NW1 1BU.
Tel: 0207 388 4097.

Diabetes

British Diabetic Association, 10 Queen Anne Street, London W1M OBD.
Tel: 0207 323 1531.

Disabled living

Disabled Living Foundation, 380–384 Harrow Road, London W9 2HU.
Tel: 0207 289 6111.

British Red Cross, 9 Grosvenor Crescent, London SW1X 7EJ.
Tel: 0207 235 5454.

Disability Scotland, Information Department, Princes House,
5 Shandwick Place, Edinburgh EH2 4RG. Tel: 0131 229 8632.

Motability, Goodman House, Station Approach, Harlow, Essex CN20 2ET.
Tel: 01279 635666.

Royal Society for Disability and Rehabilitation (RADARO), 12 City Forum,
250 City Road, London EC1V 8AF. Tel: 0207 250 3222.

Shaftesbury Society, 16 Kingston Road, London SW19 1JZ. Tel: 0208 542 5550.

Donors

National Blood Transfusion Service. Tel: 0345 71171.

National Blood Authority, Oak House, Reeds Crescent, Watford,
Herts WD1 1QH. Tel: 01923 486800. The NBA manages all NHS blood services,
including the management of the 15 regional transfusion services.

HM Inspector of Anatomy, Department of Health, Wellington House,
133–155 Waterloo Road, London SE1 8UG. Tel: 0207 972 4918.

British Organ Donor Society, Balsham, Cambridge CB1 6DL.
Tel: 01223 893636.

Down's syndrome

Down's Syndrome Association, 155 Mitcham Road, London SW17 9PG.
Tel: 0208 682 4001.

Drug addiction

National helpline. Tel: 0800 776600.

Dyslexia

British Dyslexia Association, 98 London Road, Reading, Berks RG1 5AU.
Tel: 01734 668271.

Dysphasia

Action for Dysphasic Adults, 1 Royal Street, London SE1 7LL.
Tel: 0207 261 9572

Stroke Association, Stroke House, 123–127 Whitecross Street,
London EC1Y 8JJ. Tel: 0207 489 7999.

Dystonia

Dystonia Society, 46–47 Britton Street, London EC1M 5NA. Tel: 0207 489 5671.

Eating disorders

Eating Disorders Association, First Floor, Wensum House,
103 Prince of Wales Road, Norwich NR1 1DW. Tel: 01603 619090.
Helpline: 01603 621414.

Eclampsia and pre-eclampsia

Action on Pre-eclampsia (APEC), 31–33 College Road, Harrow HA1 1EJ.
Tel: 0208 863 3271.

Eczema

see Dermatitis

Epilepsy

British Epilepsy Association, Anstey House, Hanover Square, Leeds LS3 1BE.
Tel: 0113 243 9393.

Epilepsy Association of Scotland, 48 Govan Road, Glasgow G51 1JL.
Tel: 0141 427 4911.

Family planning

Family Planning Association, 27–35 Mortimer Street, London W1N 7RG.
Tel: 0207 636 7866.

First aid

British Red Cross, 9 Grosvenor Crescent, London SW1X 7EF.
Tel: 0207 235 5454.

St John's Ambulance, 1 Grosvenor Crescent, London SW1X 7EF.
Tel: 0207 235 5231.

St Andrew's Ambulance Association, Strachan House, 16 Torphichen Street,
Edinburgh EH3 8JB. Tel: 0131 229 5419.

Haemophilia

Haemophilia Society, Chesterfield House, 385 Euston Road, London NW1 3AU.
Tel: 0207 380 0600.

Health and safety

Health and Safety Executive, 2 Southward Bridge Road, Rose Court,
London SE1 9HS. Tel: 0207 717 6104.

Health education

Health Education Authority, Trevelyan House, 30 Great Peter Street,
London SW1P 2HW. Tel: 0207 222 5300.

Huntington's chorea

Huntington's Disease Association, 108 Battersea High Street,
London SW18 3HP. Tel: 0207 223 7000.

Ileostomy

Ileostomy Association of Great Britain and Ireland, PO Box 132,
Scunthorpe DN15 9YW. Tel: 01724 720150.

Laryngectomy

National Association of Laryngectomy Clubs (NALC), Ground Floor,
6 Rickett Street, Fulham, London SW6 1RU. Tel: 0207 381 9993.

Learning disability

Mental Health Foundation, 20–21 Cornwall Terrace, London NW1 4QL.
Tel: 0207 535 7400.

British Institute of Learning Disabilities, Wolverhampton Road, Kidderminster,
Worcs DY10 3PP. Tel: 01562 850421.

MENCAP (Royal Society for Mentally Handicapped Children and Adults),
123 Golden Lane, London EC1Y 0RT. Tel: 0207 454 0454.

ENABLE (Scottish Society for the Mentally Handicapped), 7 Buchanan Street,
Glasgow G1 3HL. Tel; 0141 226 4541.

Lupus

Lupus UK, St James House, Eastern Road, Romford, Essex RM1 3NH.
Tel: 01708 731251.

Medical accidents

Action for the Victims of Medical Accidents, Bank Chambers, 1 London Road,
Forest Hill, London SE23 3TP. Tel: 0208 291 2793.

Meningitis

National Meningitis Trust, Fern House, Bath Road, Stroud GL5 3TJ.
Tel: 01453 7751738.

Mental health

MIND (National Association for Mental Health), Granta House,
15–18 Broadway, Stratford, London E15 4BQ. Tel: 0208 519 2122.

Mental Health Foundation, 20–21 Cornwall Terrace, London NW1 4QL.
Tel: 0207 535 7400.

Mental Health Act Commission, Maid Marian House, 56 Houndsgate,
Nottingham NG1 6BG. Tel: 0115 943 100.

Migraine

Migraine Action Association (British Migraine Association), 178a High Road,
Byfleet, West Byfleet, Surrey KT14 7ED. Tel: 01932 352468.

Multiple births

TAMBA (Twins and Multiple Births Association), PO Box 30, Little Sutton,
South Wirral L66 1TH. Tel: 0151 348 0020.

Multiple sclerosis

Multiple Sclerosis Society of Great Britain and Northern Ireland,
25 Effie Road, Fulham, London SW6 1EE. Tel: 0207 610 7171.

Multiple Sclerosis Resource Centre, 4a Chapel Hill, Stansted, Essex CM24 8AG.
Tel: 01279 817101.

Muscular dystrophy

Muscular Dystrophy Group of Great Britain, 71 Prescott Place,
London SW4 6BS. Tel: 0207 720 8055.

Myalgic encephalitis

ME Association, PO Box 8, 4a Corringham Road, Stanford-le-Hope, Essex SS17 OHA. Tel: 01375 361013.

Myasthenia gravis

Myasthenia Gravis Association, Keynes House, Chester Park, Alfreton Road, Derby DE21 4AS. Tel: 01332 290219.

Myopathy

see Muscular dystrophy

Narcolepsy

Narcolepsy Association (UK), 2 Bishops Close, Hurstpierpoint, Hassocks, West Sussex BN6 9XU. Tel: 01273 832725.

Nursing

Royal College of Nursing, 20 Cavendish Square, London W1M OAB. Tel: 0207 409 3333.

Osteoporosis

National Osteoporosis Society, PO Box 10, Radstock, Bath BA3 3YB. Tel: 01761 471771.

Paget's disease

National Association for the Relief of Paget's Disease, 1 Church Road, Eccles, Manchester M30 0DL. Tel: 0161 707 9225.

Paralysis

Spinal Injuries Association, 76 St James's Lane, Muswell Hill, London N10 3DF. Tel: 0208 444 2121.

Spinal Injuries Scotland, Festival Business Centre, 150 Broad Street, Glasgow G51 1DH. Tel: 0141 314 0056.

Motor Neurone Disease Association, PO Box 246, Northampton NN1 2PR. Tel: 01604 622269.

Parkinson's disease

Parkinson's Disease Society of the UK, 2215 Vauxhall Bridge Road, London SW1V 1EJ. Tel: 0207 931 8080.

Phenylketonuria

National Society for Phenylketonuria (UK) Ltd, 7 Southfield Close, Willen, Milton Keynes MK15 9LL. Tel: 0845 603 9136.

Phobias

National Phobic Society, 407 Wilbraham Road, Chorlton, Manchester M21 0UT. Tel: 0161 881 1937.

Psoriasis

National Psoriasis Association, Milton House, 7 Milton Street, Northampton NN2 7JG. Tel: 01604 711129.

Relate

National Relate, Herbert Gray College, Church Street, Rugby, Warwickshire CV21 3AP. Tel: 01788 573241.

Restricted growth

Restricted Growth Association (RGA), PO Box 18, Rugeley, Staffs WS15 2GH. Tel. 01889 576571.

Sickle-cell anaemia

Sickle Cell Society, 54 Station Road, Harlesden, London NW10 4UA. Tel: 0208 961 7795/4006.

Speech disorders

AFASIC (Unlocking Speech and Language), 347 Central Market, Smithfield, London EC1A 9NH. Tel: 0207 236 6487.

Speech therapy

Royal College of Speech and Language Therapists, 7 Bath Place, Rivington Street, London EC2A 3DR. Tel: 0207 613 3854.

Spina bifida

Association for Spina Bifida and Hydrocephalus, ASBAH House, 42 Park Road, Peterborough PE1 2U1. Tel: 01733 555988.

Scottish Spina Bifida Association, 189 Queensferry Road, Edinburgh EH4 2BW. Tel: 0131 332 0743.

Sudden heart death syndrome

Foundation for the Study of Sudden Heart Deaths, 14 Halkin Street, London SW1X 7DP. Tel: 0207 235 0965.

Talking books

Calibre, Aylesbury, Bucks HP22 5XQ. Tel: 01296 432339.

Listening Books, 12 Lant Street, London SE1 1QH. Tel: 0207 407 9417.

Tinnitus

see Deafness

Toy libraries

National Association of Toy and Leisure Libraries/Playmatters, 68 Churchway, London NW1 1LT. Tel: 0207 387 9592.

Turner's syndrome

UK Turner Syndrome Society, c/o Child Growth Foundation, 2 Mayfield Avenue, London W4 1PW. Tel: 0208 995 0257.

Voluntary organisations

National Council for Voluntary Organisations, Regents Wharf, 8 All Saints Street, London N1 9RL. Tel: 0207 713 6161.

Measurements in medicine

SI units commonly used in medicine

Quantity	SI unit (abbreviation)
Length	Metre (m)
Area	Square metre (m^2)
Volume	Cubic metric (m^3) = 100 litres (L)
Mass	Kilogram (kg)
Amount of substance	Mole (mol)
Energy	Joule (J)
Pressure	Pascal (Pa)
Force	Newton (N)
Time	Second (s)
Frequency	Hertz (Hz)
Power	Watt (w)
Temperature	Degree Celsius (°C)

Multiples and submultiples

Factor	Prefix	Abbreviation
10^6	Mega-	M
10^3	Kilo-	k
10^{-1}	Deci-	d
10^{-2}	Centi-	c
10^{-3}	Milli-	m
10^{-6}	Micro-	
10^{-9}	Nano-	n
10^{-12}	Pico-	p

International organisations

World Health Organisation (WHO)

Founded in 1948, the WHO is a United Nations Agency whose objectives are to attain the highest possible level of health worldwide and to eradicate infectious disease through vaccination programmes.

The organisation is based in Geneva with an office in each of its six regions, usually in the ministry of health.

Its functions include the following:

- setting standards in healthcare
- advocating health policy reform
- working closely with governments in the areas of maternal and child health, populations, planning, nutrition, sanitation, and the supply and distribution of medicines.

Policy is set out at the Annual General Meeting of the World Assembly, which is attended by representatives from member states. The WHO is headed by its director general, who is supported by administrative, technical and medical staff.

The WHO has been successful in the eradication of smallpox, with the last reported case occurring in 1977.

World Medical Association (WMA)

The WMA is an independent confederation of non-governmental professional medical associations from around the world, founded in 1947. The association is non-political and provides a forum for member associations to communicate with each other and to achieve consensus.

The WMA promotes the following:

- high standards of professional medical care and ethics

- professional freedom of physicians thereby facilitating high-calibre medical care.

Since its foundation, and through its declarations, the WMA has developed guidance for doctors, national medical associations, governments and other international bodies. The areas covered include patients' rights, research on humane subjects, torture of prisoners, use and misuse of drugs, family planning and the care of sick and wounded people in times of conflict.

Commonwealth Medical Association (CMA)

The Commonwealth Medical Association is a non-governmental body that has a good working relationship with both the World Health Organisation and the health aspects of the United Nations.

The CMA is based in the UK and is subscribed to by a number of national medical associations.

The CMA's main objectives are as follows:

- to strengthen the capacity of national medical associations by collaborating with other health professional associations
- to improve the health status of vulnerable and disadvantaged groups in developing countries.

The main activities of the Association are in the fields of women's, young people's and sexual health. It is also concerned with the ethical and human rights implications of providing health information and services.

Professional organisations relating to complementary medicine

Acupuncture

British Medical Acupuncture Society, Newton House, Newton Lane, Whitley, Warrington WA4 4JA. Tel: 01925 730727.

British Acupuncture Council, Park House, 206–208 Latimer Road, London W10 6RE. Tel: 0208 964 0222.

Alexander technique

Society of Teachers of the Alexander Technique, 20 London House, 266 Fulham Road, London SW10 8EL. Tel: 0207 351 0828.

Aromatherapy

Aromatherapy Organisations Council, 3 Latymer Close, Braybrooke, Market Harborough LE16 9LN. Tel: 01858 434242.

Chiropractic

British Chiropractic Association, 29 Whitley Street, Reading, Berkshire RG2 03G. Tel: 01734 757557.

Chiropractic Patients Association, 8 Centre One, Lysander Way, Old Sarum Park, Salisbury, Wilts SP4 6BU. Tel: 01722 415027.

Homeopathy

British Homeopathic Association, 271 Devonshire Street, London WIN 1RJ. Tel: 0207 935 2163.

Faculty of Homeopathy, 2 Powis Place, Great Ormond Street,
London WC1N 3HT. Tel: 0207 837 9469.

Hydrotherapy

Chartered Society of Physiotherapists, 14 Bedford Row, London WC1R 4ED.
Tel: 0207 306 6666.

Hypnotherapy

British Society of Medical and Dental Hypnosis, 17 Keppel View Road,
Kimberworth, Rotherham, Yorkshire S61 2AR. Tel: 01709 554558.

National School of Hypnotherapy and Psychotherapy, The Central Register of
Advanced Hypnotherapists, 28 Finsbury Park Road, London N4 2JX.
Tel: 0207 359 6991.

Osteopathy

General Council and Register of Osteopaths, 56 London Street, Reading,
Berks RG1 4SQ. Tel: 01734 576585.

Reflexology

Association of Reflexologists, 27 Old Gloucester Street, London WC1 3XX.
Tel: 0870 5673320.

British Reflexology Association, Monks Orchard, Whitbourne,
Worcs WR6 5RB. Tel: 01886 821207.

Index

£20·80